T0333956

THE **NURSE'S** GUIDE TO

MENTAL HEALTH MEDICINES

Sara Miller McCune founded SAGE Publishing in 1965 to support the dissemination of usable knowledge and educate a global community. SAGE publishes more than 1000 journals and over 800 new books each year, spanning a wide range of subject areas. Our growing selection of library products includes archives, data, case studies and video. SAGE remains majority owned by our founder and after her lifetime will become owned by a charitable trust that secures the company's continued independence.

Los Angeles | London | New Delhi | Singapore | Washington DC | Melbourne

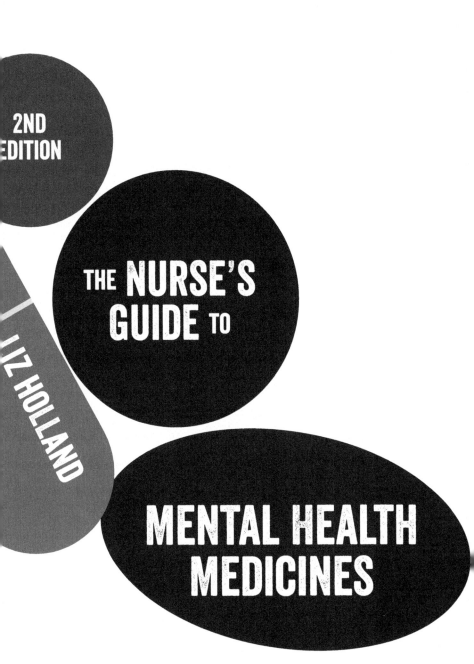

2ND EDITION

LIZ HOLLAND

THE **NURSE'S GUIDE** TO

MENTAL HEALTH MEDICINES

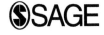

SAGE

Los Angeles | London | New Delhi
Singapore | Washington DC | Melbourne

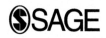

Los Angeles | London | New Delhi
Singapore | Washington DC | Melbourne

SAGE Publications Ltd
1 Oliver's Yard
55 City Road
London EC1Y 1SP

SAGE Publications Inc.
2455 Teller Road
Thousand Oaks, California 91320

SAGE Publications India Pvt Ltd
B 1/I 1 Mohan Cooperative Industrial Area
Mathura Road
New Delhi 110 044

SAGE Publications Asia-Pacific Pte Ltd
3 Church Street
#10-04 Samsung Hub
Singapore 049483

Editor: Alex Clabburn
Assistant editor: Ruth Lilly
Production editor: Martin Fox
Copyeditor: William Baginsky
Proofreader: Elaine Leek
Indexer: Gary Kirby
Marketing manager: Ruslana Khatagova
Cover design: Sheila Tong
Typeset by: C&M Digitals (P) Ltd, Chennai, India
Printed in the UK

Library of Congress Control Number: 2021945517

British Library Cataloguing in Publication data

A catalogue record for this book is available from
the British Library

ISBN 978-1-5297-6903-6
ISBN 978-1-5297-6902-9 (pbk)

At SAGE we take sustainability seriously. Most of our products are printed in the UK using responsibly
sourced papers and boards. When we print overseas we ensure sustainable papers are used as
measured by the PREPS grading system. We undertake an annual audit to monitor our sustainability.

CONTENTS

ABOUT THE AUTHOR AND CONTRIBUTORS

Liz Holland is a registered mental health nurse (RMN) and experienced NHS leader, currently working as an NHS director. Liz became a mental health nurse after completing a PGDip in Mental Health Nursing at King's College London. Prior to her nurse training, Liz gained a BSc (Hons) in Psychology with Mental and Physical Healthcare from the University of Reading. Liz also has an MSc in Psychosocial Interventions from Kingston and St George's University and an MBA from the University of Brighton.

Emily Floyd is an experienced RMN and has worked across several challenging acute inpatient environments. Emily has been part of award-winning nursing teams, and also has an expertise and interest in spirituality and mental health. She has a BA (Hons) from King's College London in the Study of Religions alongside her BSc in Mental Health Nursing, also obtained from King's College London, and has undertaken considerable post-registration training, particularly in relation to complex physical healthcare. Emily is also a graduate of the NHS Leadership Academy and continues to develop and build on her skills as a passionate member of the frontline NHS workforce. Emily is currently working in the NHS as a quality improvement specialist.

Sara Soames graduated from the University of Manchester in 2012 with a BSc in Mental Health Nursing. Having loved her older adult experience as a student nurse, she knew that this was the field in which she would eventually specialise. Following a short spell on an acute working-age adult ward, she took up a role as a deputy ward manager on an older person's mental health ward, where her passion for improving the quality of life of older people with mental health illnesses and supporting their carers flourished. She has since worked as a care coordinator in the community and dementia nurse specialist in a memory assessment service, before becoming a pathway lead for older adult mental health services. In the future, Sara hopes to complete a master's degree, and would be interested in conducting research into the effects of a dementia diagnosis in those who have a pre-existing diagnosis of emotionally unstable or borderline personality disorder.

AUTHOR ACKNOWLEDGEMENTS

Thank you to SAGE Publications for giving us the opportunity to create this book, and thank you, in particular, to Alex Clabburn, Ruth Lilly, Charlène Burin and Becky Taylor, as their hard work and support has made the initial idea to create this book become a reality and progress to a second edition.

ABOUT THE BOOK

Welcome to *The Nurse's Guide to Mental Health Medicines*, second edition! This book has been developed as a simple and easy-to-read guide that outlines some of the most frequently used medicines in mental health treatment and provides some suggestions on how best to support people taking these medicines (or know what support you may need, if you are using these medicines yourself).

It is important to point out that this book is not designed as a 'prescriber's guide', and it is not designed to replace regulated guidance on medicines and dosing, such as the British National Formulary (BNF). This book should be used as a reference guide and information source, but before initiating any pharmacological treatment, it is highly recommended that medical and pharmaceutical advice is sought and that the BNF is checked, and local organisational policies and procedures are consulted and followed at all times.

All the people who have contributed to this book are currently registered mental health nurses who are active in clinical mental health settings. The information that they write in their chapters is based on their own experiences. All the case studies mentioned in the book are based on real clinical experiences, but details and names have been changed so as to ensure that confidentiality is respected at all times.

This book will use and reference evidence-based best practice and research in all the chapters, but it will also use and signpost to less academic sources such as blog sites and resources developed by charitable organisations specialising in mental health. This is because the book is not just about sharing the guidance around medicines best practice; it seeks to share how people truly feel about mental health and mental health medicines, value the perspective of people with lived experience, and signpost mental health professionals to resources and to information that is appropriate and accessible in format that can be used in their daily clinical practice. Any text that is not referenced is the opinion of the author of the chapter, based on their clinical knowledge.

This book has been written as it was felt that although there are many complex and comprehensive textbooks available on pharmacology, a plethora of research and journal articles available at the touch of a button and information such as the BNF that can be used as an aid to prescribing treatment, there was not a simple and easy-to-read guide that a busy member of nursing staff could read through in order to refresh or enhance their knowledge, or that a student nurse new to pharmacology could look at to get a flavour of this complex and vast subject. Similarly, this book may help those using mental health medicines and their family and friend carers to feel more confident in their understanding of medications and know what questions to ask and what support to look for. Overall, it is hoped that this book increases awareness of medication and gets people talking about medicines!

The book is suitable for everyone and anyone, but has been written with nurses, student nurses and nursing assistants particularly in mind. The message of the book is that all content is like a handover: a sharing of knowledge 'by nurses, for nurses'. The content is also suitable for people who are using mental health services and would like to develop their knowledge around mental health medicines, and for the families, friends and carers of people using mental health services.

Each chapter includes ideas on how to explore the subject further. It sets out clear objectives at the start of the chapter, detailing what it will help the reader to achieve, and has a summary of learning and a section on references and recommended reading at the end. Each chapter (other than Chapter 7, which is already age group specific) includes a section on how the topic applies to children, young people and older adults. Unless otherwise stated, the definition we are using of an older adult is a person over 65 years of age. Each chapter also includes information on key medicines that may be used in the specialism that the chapter covers and brings all the learning from the chapter together and applies the information to a case scenario. The Glossary at the end of the book provides explanations of words highlighted in bold in the text.

The book covers the most pertinent areas in which mental health medications may be used, but there may be other individual situations and needs for medicines that are not covered here. The book also does not include an exhaustive list of all medicines used in mental health. The clinicians who have been involved in the production of this book have selected the medicines that they have most used in their clinical experience to date to discuss in their chapters.

Nearly everyone who is reading this book will have taken some form of medication in their life, whether it was for a physical or a mental health illness, and so we can all relate to the experience of being started on a new treatment; having an unfamiliar box of pills; worrying about a list of side effects that sound, frankly, terrifying! Those of us working as health professionals therefore have a responsibility to support people in our care who need medication to make this feel a safe and supportive experience, and it is hoped that this book will help health professionals and people using mental health services, and their families, friends and carers, to feel empowered to discuss medicines openly. In the world of medicines, knowledge is always power.

I really hope that you enjoy the book and that you find it useful.

Liz Holland

1 ANTIDEPRESSANT MEDICATIONS

LIZ HOLLAND

AFTER READING THIS CHAPTER, YOU WILL BE ABLE TO:

- Consider the needs of individuals who may take antidepressant medication
- Have a basic awareness of how antidepressant medications came about
- Hold a basic understanding of the different types of antidepressant medications and how they work
- Consider the risks and benefits of different types of antidepressant medications
- Apply basic knowledge around antidepressant medications to clinical decision-making

WHEN DO WE NEED ANTIDEPRESSANT MEDICATIONS?

Since the 1980s, depression has been referred to as the 'common cold' of mental illness (Rottmann, 1986) due to its high prevalence rate. Many people in the UK have been affected by depression in some way, whether it be because they have lived the experience of depression themselves or because they have seen a friend or family member battle an episode of depression. Office for National Statistics (ONS) data from March 2021 indicated that around 21 per cent of adults in the UK were showing clinical symptoms of depression.

Depression is a mood disorder and is characterised by symptoms such as: feelings of helplessness and hopelessness, a loss of interest in daily activities and a feeling of having no energy, disruption to sleep and appetite, having difficulties in being able to concentrate, negative thinking and having thoughts of guilt and worthlessness.

Living with depression can be incredibly debilitating for people, and the following blog entry demonstrates the daily struggles that people living with depression can face.

Stepped into the black hole. i don't know why. i don't know

when. this was not on the schedule. i was not prepared.

heavy. hurts to stand. hurts to sit. breathing takes all the

energy i've got. nothing poetic or dramatic to say. can't

breathe. can't think. brain is not my own. thoughts of

nonsense. focus – i have none. never will be able to explain

the whole-body experience of crippling depression. never. i

can feel the hole in the middle of my chest ...

(Etta 2008, published in Kotliar, 2016: 1206)

In severe cases of depression, sufferers can experience thoughts of suicidality; some individuals may feel that they need to act on these, and approximately 15 per cent of people with depression go on to die from suicide (Jiaquan Xu et al., 2016).

The causes of depression are still not fully understood. However, there is a generally accepted argument that there is some level of biological influence, although this is in conjunction with other psychological and sociological factors.

The biological explanation of depression is based on the role of three **neurotransmitters** in the brain: serotonin, dopamine and norepinephrine. Neurotransmitters are chemical messengers for the brain; they help different areas of the brain communicate with one another. Serotonin, dopamine and norepinephrine are particularly important in the areas of mood, sexual desire and sexual function, sleep, memory, appetite and social behaviour. Therefore, it makes sense that, as these are the areas in which people experience difficulties when they have an episode of depression, the neurotransmitters linked to them may also be involved in the depression. However, the biological explanation proposed for depression was only suggested after the invention of antidepressants, rather than before. Indeed, antidepressants and their effects on mood were initially discovered by accident, and there is still only a very limited understanding of why and how they work. For some people, they just do!

Since the 1950s, when antidepressants first became available on the commercial market, it has been suggested that depression is caused by an imbalance in the levels of these neurotransmitters in the brain, in particular of serotonin (prior to this, stimulant drugs were given to people with depression!). However, there is little scientific evidence to support this. It is currently being suggested that people who are vulnerable to depression have less sensitive serotonin receptors in their brain than those who are not vulnerable to depression (Kring et al., 2013). This means that people who are vulnerable to depression may not be able to produce as much serotonin in their brains, and this goes on to affect their mood and behaviour.

There are four different types of antidepressant medication and, although the mechanisms that enable each of these types to work are slightly different, overall the common theme with all antidepressants is that they enable the levels of serotonin, dopamine and norepinephrine to rise in the brain, and these increased levels seem to lead to an improvement in symptoms for some people. However, it should be noted that this explanation is limited: we know that the increased levels of neurotransmitters in the brain occur merely hours after a dose of an antidepressant medication is ingested, yet, typically, antidepressants take about two to six weeks to have a noticeable effect; there is currently no convincing biological explanation for this.

The four different categories of antimedications and the intricacies of how they work will now be discussed.

WHAT ARE THE DIFFERENT TYPES OF ANTIDEPRESSANT MEDICATIONS AND HOW DO THEY WORK?

The earliest category of antidepressant medications came onto the commercial market in 1957 (Moncrieff, 2011) and these are known as tricyclic antidepressants. You may recognise names such as imipramine and amitriptyline, which are the most well-known and well-used drugs of the tricyclic family. Most simply, the tricyclics cause the brain to increase the production of serotonin and norepinephrine, alongside stopping the production of another neurotransmitter known as acetylcholine, which in high levels is known to inhibit serotonin production. However, problems with tricyclic antidepressants were quickly identified: they had serious toxic effects on the cardiac systems of some individuals and were also highly toxic if they were taken even in small amounts in overdose situations, which is not ideal when they are being prescribed for a client group who may be experiencing thoughts of ending their life.

Monoamine oxidase inhibitor (MAOI) antidepressants were the next type of antidepressant to arrive. They were developed because they had less severe side effects than those of the tricyclics and were also noted to be very good at treating feelings of anxiety as well as the symptoms of depression. MAOIs work by preventing the breakdown of serotonin and norepinephrine in the brain, thus leading to increased levels of these neurotransmitters within the brain. The most concerning side effect of MAOIs is their impact on blood pressure: they are linked to the development of **postural hypotension**, particularly in older people. Something important to note is that people on MAOI antidepressants must follow a strict diet and avoid any food or drink products that contain tyramine (see Fact Box 1.1). If tyramine is consumed by someone who is taking an MAOI, it can cause a severe headache and a sudden increase in blood pressure, known as a **hypertensive** crisis. Over-the-counter medicines that can be used to treat coughs and colds can also cause sudden hypertensive crisis in people who are taking MAOIs so it is important to talk to a doctor, nurse or pharmacist before such medication is taken.

Today, MAOIs and tricyclics are less likely to be used than the selective serotonin reuptake inhibitor (SSRI) antidepressants (below) as they have more severe side effects. They are more often used in older people, or in people with depression who have not responded to SSRI medication.

FACT BOX 1.1

What sorts of foods contain tyramine?

- Cheese
- Alcohol and non-alcoholic beer
- Gravy
- Salami, pepperoni and other cured meats
- Marmite
- Yoghurt
- Oxo
- Bovril
- Liver
- Chocolate
- Foods that are beginning to go off

SSRIs and serotonin and norepinephrine reuptake inhibitors (SNRIs) are the final two types of antidepressants and are the most modern. In general, they are noted to have fewer side effects than the older tricyclics and MAOIs.

SSRIs are medicines that work specifically on the neurotransmitter serotonin. They prevent the reuptake of serotonin within the brain, which allows levels of serotonin to build up. SSRIs are the most common type of antidepressant used and tend to be the first-line medicinal intervention.

SNRIs are the newest type of antidepressant available. They work by preventing the reuptake of both serotonin and norepinephrine within the brain, thus leading to increased levels. They are less commonly used than SSRIs and may be used in more difficult situations to treat cases of depression.

These two kinds of antidepressant medications have similar side effect profiles due to their similar mechanisms of action. Neither of these types of antidepressants are recommended for use in under-18s as they can increase feelings of suicidality. These medicines can interact with herbal remedies, in particular St John's wort.

For both the SSRIs and the SNRIs, the most common side effects are gastrointestinal upsets, dizziness, feelings of anxiety and shakiness, a dry mouth, headaches and **sexual dysfunction**. Some patients refer to these feelings as being a little bit like 'having a really horrible hangover'.

This is only a brief summary of the different types of antidepressants and how they work. If you would like to read about this in more detail and/or would like to look more at how neurotransmitters work within the brain, please see the References and Recommended Reading list at the end of each chapter of this book.

It may be of interest to know that the current NICE (National Institute for Health and Care Excellence) recommendation on antidepressants for adults is that an SSRI should be the first-line medication to be offered and tried as overall they have the best risk–benefit ratio, and sertraline should be the first drug of choice as this is the most cost-effective (NICE, 2016).

Serotonin syndrome

It is very important to be aware of a potentially fatal condition known as 'serotonin syndrome' that can occur in people who are taking antidepressants. It is particularly linked with SSRI antidepressants and occurs when the levels of serotonin in the brain become too high. It is more likely to occur in patients who are taking two different types of antidepressant together. The initial symptoms of serotonin syndrome include:

- Sweating and shivering
- Feeling agitated and/or confused
- Diarrhoea
- Muscle spasms or twitching.

All patients taking antidepressants should be made aware of these symptoms, and if they are experienced, patients should immediately contact their GP or mental health professional.

Occasionally, serotonin syndrome may become severe and this is when it can be life-threatening if treatment is not sought. Alongside the symptoms listed above, severe cases of serotonin syndrome will include:

- Seizures
- Fever (marked by a very high temperature, over 38°C)
- Drowsiness or total loss of consciousness
- Irregular heartbeat.

These symptoms are a medical emergency and so 999 treatment must be immediately sought. When working with patients who take antidepressant medication and with their friends and families, it is important to discuss serotonin syndrome openly and to make sure that if emergency treatment for serotonin syndrome is needed, then they know to inform the treating practitioners that the person is on an antidepressant medication, and that they inform them of the name and dose of the medication, alongside any other medicines that the person is taking.

Withdrawal syndrome

No matter what type of antidepressant medication someone is taking, it is really important that medication is not suddenly stopped in the middle of treatment. This can be dangerous and can make the person stopping the medicine feel really unwell. We call this 'withdrawal syndrome'. For this reason, if a decision is reached that a person is going to stop taking their antidepressant medication, it is really important that a plan is made to gradually reduce the dose, rather than suddenly cease all medication. A person can develop withdrawal symptoms even when there is a careful plan in place to slowly reduce the medication, but they are less likely to be severe. Also, by having a plan in place, the person will see a health professional regularly, which allows for close monitoring and regular discussion about how the person is feeling.

All the different types of antidepressant medicines can lead to withdrawal symptoms, and the reaction that someone has to coming off their medicine is unique to them as an individual. Interestingly, research by the Royal College of Psychiatrists (2014) shows that venlafaxine is the drug most likely to cause severe withdrawal effects, and that 82 per cent of those coming off venlafaxine suffer from some level of withdrawal symptoms. Typically, withdrawal symptoms seemed to occur for six to eight weeks following the discontinuation of medication.

The Royal College of Psychiatrists (2014) found that the most common withdrawal symptom for patients coming off antidepressants was increased feelings of anxiety, with 70 per cent noting this experience. Other common withdrawal symptoms include:

- Finding it hard to sleep
- Increasing feelings of low mood and/or thoughts of suicide
- Feeling dizzy
- Disturbing and/or vivid dreams
- Headaches
- Sickness and stomach upsets
- Flu-like symptoms
- Feeling like an electric shock is passing through your body.

GO FURTHER ...

If you would like to download some simple and easy to understand fact sheets around antidepressants, the two links below are helpful:

www.rcpsych.ac.uk/mental-health/treatments-and-wellbeing/antidepressants

www.mind.org.uk/information-support/drugs-and-treatments/antidepressants/about-antidepressants

WHAT OTHER IMPORTANT INFORMATION AROUND ANTIDEPRESSANTS DO I NEED TO MAKE SURE THAT I TALK ABOUT WITH PEOPLE TAKING THE MEDICATION?

- For anyone who is taking an MAOI, you need to ensure that they understand the information around diet restrictions and cough/cold medications. People on MAOIs carry a patient information card with these details: ensure that they have this card, that they understand the information and that they carry it somewhere safe. In inpatient services, a dietician should always be contacted for a patient on an MAOI in order to have a safe, personalised meal plan created.
- When you are working with someone who is taking any kind of antidepressant medication, it is really important that you talk about the side effects that they are experiencing. Even side effects that you may think

of as 'mild' can be incredibly debilitating for people and may cause them to stop taking their medication. There is a brilliant tool that was created by the Royal College of Psychiatrists in 2009, which you can download for free to help you structure and record these discussions. It is called the Antidepressant Side Effect Checklist (ASEC) and can be completed by a patient and health professional together. It would also be helpful to have a family, friend or carer of the patient present if they would like.

- As nurses, we need to talk about sex! Sexual side effects can be incredibly debilitating for people taking antidepressants and can actually cause patients to stop taking their medication. These sexual side effects are severe; for example, fluoxetine is actually also prescribed as a treatment for premature ejaculation in males, such does it delay ejaculation. Unfortunately, research shows that the main barrier to discussions around sex is the anxiety of the nurse (Gott et al., 2004), and so it is really important that we get over this barrier and encourage open discussions around all aspects of a person's health.

GO FURTHER ...

If you would like to read more information around the development of the ASEC tool discussed above (Uher et al. on behalf of the Royal College of Psychiatrists, 2009) please visit: http://bjp.rcpsych.org/content/195/3/202.full-text.pdf+html where the full article can be obtained. A copy of the ASEC tool can be downloaded from the appendices section of the article.

THE MEDICINES LIST

This medicines list will look at the most commonly used medicines for depression in mental health services, and these medicines will be categorised into tricyclics, MAOIs, SSRIs and SNRIs. The chemical name and UK brand name of each drug will be given, the average doses, and any important contraindications to be aware of. A brief side effects profile is given for each drug category. This is not an exhaustive list of all antidepressant medications. You can download a list of all antidepressants and their properties that are currently being used in the UK at: www.mind.org.uk/information-support/drugs-and-treatments/antidepressants-a-z/overview if required. Remember, as a nurse, you are responsible for knowing and understanding every medicine that you dispense and administer to a patient (NMC, 2020).

Tricyclic antidepressants

The side effect profile for tricyclics

The most common side effects of tricyclics include: feelings of increased anxiety, **constipation**, dry mouth, problems urinating, increased agitation, blurred vision, drowsiness, shaky hands, low blood pressure, diarrhoea, feeling confused, feeling very hungry, reduced appetite, feeling sick, finding it hard to sleep, feelings of pins and needles, feeling restless, nightmares, reduced sexual desire, finding it hard to reach sexual orgasm, stomach cramps, a funny taste in the mouth. Rare side effects can include seizures, blood disorders, problems with the liver, heart attacks and strokes.

Drug name: **Amitriptyline**

UK brand names: None known

Average doses: 75–200mg per day

What form does it come in? Liquid and tablet

Does it interact with any other medicines? Yes. The following interactions are known:

- *Sleeping tablets and tranquillisers:* It is known that amitriptyline can increase the sedative effects of any medicine that makes you sleepy
- *Antipsychotic medicines (particularly typical antipsychotics):* Taking amitriptyline alongside an antipsychotic drug can increase the risk of developing a problem with the rhythm of the heart
- *MAOI antidepressants:* Severe side effects are more common if amitriptyline is taken in conjunction with an MAOI

(Continued)

- *SSRI antidepressants*: If an SSRI is taken alongside amitriptyline, the level of the SSRI drug can become higher than expected within the body, and this can cause serious side effects
- *St John's wort*: You are at an increased risk of developing serotonin syndrome if you take amitriptyline alongside St John's wort. It can also affect the efficacy of amitriptyline

Drug name: Clomipramine

UK brand names: Anafranil

Average doses: 10-250mg per day

What form does it come in? Capsule and slow release tablet

Does it interact with any other medicines? Yes. The following interactions are known:

- *Sleeping tablets and tranquillisers*: It is known that clomipramine can increase the sedative effects of any medicine that makes you sleepy
- *Antipsychotic medicines (particularly typical antipsychotics)*: Taking clomipramine alongside an antipsychotic can increase the risk of developing a problem with the rhythm of the heart
- *MAOI antidepressants*: Severe side effects are more common if you take clomipramine in conjunction with an MAOI
- *SSRI antidepressants*: If you take an SSRI alongside clomipramine, the level of the SSRI drug can become higher than expected within the body, and this can cause serious side effects
- *St John's wort*: You are at an increased risk of developing serotonin syndrome if you take clomipramine alongside St John's wort. It can also affect the efficacy of clomipramine

Drug name: Imipramine

UK brand names: Tofranil

Average doses: 75-200mg per day

What form does it come in? Liquid and tablet

Does it interact with any other medicines? Yes. The following interactions are known:

- *Sleeping tablets and tranquillisers*: It is known that imipramine can increase the sedative effects of any medicine that makes you sleepy
- *Antipsychotic medicines (particularly typical antipsychotics)*: Taking imipramine alongside an antipsychotic can increase the risk of developing a problem with the rhythm of the heart
- *MAOI antidepressants*: Severe side effects are more common if you take imipramine in conjunction with an MAOI
- *SSRI antidepressants*: If you take an SSRI alongside imipramine, the level of the SSRI drug can become higher than expected within the body, and this can cause serious side effects
- *St John's wort*: You are at an increased risk of developing serotonin syndrome if you take imipramine alongside St John's wort. It can also affect the efficacy of imipramine

MAOIs

The side effect profile for MAOIs

The most common side effects for MAOIs include: finding it hard to sleep, dry mouth, feeling exhausted, headaches, vomiting, feeling sick, dizziness, blurred vision, twitching, muscle spasms and jerks, diarrhoea, and postural hypotension. This is in addition to the dietary modifications discussed above. Rare side effects can include jaundice, liver damage, blood disorders, glaucoma, a lupus-like illness and **hallucinations**.

Drug name: **Phenelzine**

UK brand names: Nardil

Average doses: 15–45mg per day

(Continued)

What form does it come in? Tablet only

Does it interact with any other medicines? Yes. The following interactions are known:

- *Carbamazepine*: If you take carbamazepine alongside phenelzine this can reduce the levels of phenelzine in your blood, which makes it less effective
- *Clozapine*: Taking clozapine alongside phenelzine can increase the effect of the phenelzine on the brain, which may then worsen side effects
- *Tricyclic antidepressants*: Phenelzine is known to have poor interaction with any of the tricyclic antidepressants so combining the two should be avoided
- *SSRI and SNRI antidepressants*: Phenelzine is known to have poor interaction with any of the SSRI and SNRI antidepressants so combining these should be avoided
- *St John's wort*: You are at an increased risk of developing serotonin syndrome if you take phenelzine alongside St John's wort. It can also affect the efficacy of phenelzine

Drug name: Tranylcypromine

UK brand names: Parnate

Average doses: 20–30mg per day. This should always be split into two doses, and both of these doses need to be taken on separate occasions before 3 p.m.

What form does it come in? Tablet only

Does it interact with any other medicines? Yes. The following interactions are known:

- *Carbamazepine*: If you take carbamazepine alongside tranylcypromine this can reduce the levels of tranylcypromine in your blood, which then makes it less effective
- *Clozapine*: Taking clozapine alongside tranylcypromine can increase the effect of the tranylcypromine on the brain, which may then worsen side effects

- *Tricyclic antidepressants*: Tranylcypromine is known to have poor interaction with any of the tricyclic antidepressants so combining the two should be avoided
- *SSRI and SNRI antidepressants*: Tranylcypromine is known to have poor interaction with any of the SSRI and SNRI antidepressants so combining these should be avoided
- *St John's wort*: You are at an increased risk of developing serotonin syndrome if you take tranylcypromine alongside St John's wort. It can also affect the efficacy of tranylcypromine

SSRIs

The side effect profile for SSRIs

The most common side effects of SSRIs include: a loss of energy, headaches, feeling sick, difficulties sleeping, feeling very tired, sweating more, a dry mouth, feeling drowsy, constipation, diarrhoea, feeling more anxious, shaky hands, vomiting, achy muscles and joints, stomach cramps, stuffy nose, loss of appetite, reduced sexual desire, finding it hard to reach sexual orgasm, distorted taste, dizziness, feeling itchy, feeling more agitated, lots of saliva in the mouth. Rare side effects can include fainting, hair loss, very heavy periods in women, seizures, liver problems, blood disorders, nosebleeds, tooth-grinding and panic attacks.

Drug name: **Citalopram**

UK brand names: Cipramil

Average doses: 20–40mg per day

What form does it come in? Oral drops and tablet

Does it interact with any other medicines? Yes. The following interactions are known:

(Continued)

- *Carbamazepine*: If you take carbamazepine alongside citalopram this can reduce the levels of citalopram in your blood, which then makes it less effective
- *Antipsychotic medicines*: Typical antipsychotics interact with citalopram and increase the risk of developing a problem with the rhythm of the heart. Taking clozapine alongside citalopram can lead to an increase in clozapine levels
- *MAOI antidepressants*: Serotonin syndrome is more likely if you take citalopram alongside an MAOI
- *Tricyclic antidepressants*: Taking citalopram alongside a tricyclic antidepressant can increase the levels of the tricyclic antidepressant in the blood, and this may then lead to increased side effects
- *St John's wort*: You are at an increased risk of developing serotonin syndrome if you take citalopram and St John's wort together. St John's wort can also affect the efficacy of citalopram

---

Drug name: **Escitalopram**

UK brand names: Cipralex

Average doses: 10–20mg per day

What form does it come in? Oral drops and tablet

Does it interact with any other medicines? Yes. The following interactions are known:

- *Antipsychotic medicines (typical)*: Typical antipsychotics interact with escitalopram and increase the risk of developing a problem with the rhythm of the heart
- *MAOI antidepressants*: Serotonin syndrome is more likely if you take escitalopram alongside an MAOI
- *Tricyclic antidepressants*: Taking escitalopram alongside a tricyclic antidepressant can increase the levels of the tricyclic antidepressant in the blood, and this may then lead to increased side effects
- *St John's wort*: You are at an increased risk of developing serotonin syndrome if you take escitalopram and St John's wort together. St John's wort can also affect the efficacy of escitalopram

Drug name: **Fluoxetine**

UK brand names: Prozac, Prozep, Oxactin

Average doses: 20mg per day

What form does it come in? Liquid and capsule

Does it interact with any other medicines? Yes. The following interactions are known:

- *Carbamazepine*: If you take carbamazepine alongside fluoxetine this can reduce the levels of fluoxetine in your blood, which then makes it less effective
- *Antipsychotic medicines*: Typical antipsychotics interact with fluoxetine and can increase the risk of developing a problem with the rhythm of the heart. Taking clozapine alongside fluoxetine can lead to an increase in clozapine levels. Taking fluoxetine alongside aripiprazole can lead to an increase in aripiprazole levels
- *MAOI antidepressants*: Serotonin syndrome is more likely if you take fluoxetine alongside an MAOI
- *Tricyclic antidepressants*: Taking fluoxetine alongside a tricyclic antidepressant can increase the levels of the tricyclic antidepressant in the blood, and this may then lead to increased side effects
- *Mirtazapine*: In addition, it has been noted that taking the combination of fluoxetine and mirtazapine can cause severe side effects
- *St John's wort*: You are at an increased risk of developing serotonin syndrome if you take fluoxetine and St John's wort together. St John's wort can also affect the efficacy of fluoxetine

Drug name: **Paroxetine**

UK brand names: Seroxat

Average doses: 20–50mg per day

What form does it come in? Liquid and tablet

Does it interact with any other medicines? Yes. The following interactions are known:

(Continued)

- *Carbamazepine*: If you take carbamazepine alongside paroxetine this can reduce the levels of paroxetine in your blood, which then makes it less effective
- *Antipsychotic medicines*: Typical antipsychotics interact with paroxetine and increase the risk of developing a problem with the rhythm of the heart. Taking clozapine alongside paroxetine can lead to an increase in clozapine levels. Taking paroxetine alongside aripiprazole can lead to an increase in aripiprazole levels
- *MAOI antidepressants*: Serotonin syndrome is more likely if you take paroxetine alongside an MAOI
- *Tricyclic antidepressants*: Taking paroxetine alongside a tricyclic antidepressant can increase the levels of the tricyclic antidepressant in the blood, and this may then lead to increased side effects
- *St John's wort*: You are at an increased risk of developing serotonin syndrome if you take paroxetine and St John's wort together. St John's wort can also affect the efficacy of paroxetine

***Drug name*: Sertraline**

UK brand names: Lustral

Average doses: 50-200mg per day

What form does it come in? Tablet only

Does it interact with any other medicines? Yes. The following interactions are known:

- *Carbamazepine*: If you take carbamazepine alongside sertraline, this can reduce the levels of sertraline in your blood, which then makes it less effective
- *Antipsychotic medicines*: Typical antipsychotics interact with sertraline and can increase the risk of developing a problem with the rhythm of the heart. Taking clozapine alongside sertraline can lead to an increase in clozapine levels
- *MAOI antidepressants*: Serotonin syndrome is more likely if you take sertraline alongside an MAOI

- *Tricyclic antidepressants*: Taking sertraline alongside a tricyclic antidepressant can increase the levels of the tricyclic antidepressant in the blood, and this may then lead to increased side effects
- *St John's wort*: You are at an increased risk of developing serotonin syndrome if you take sertraline and St John's wort together. St John's wort can also affect the efficacy of sertraline

SNRIs

The side effect profile for SNRIs

The most common side effects for SNRIs include: increasing sweating, night sweats, headaches, dry mouth, dizziness, feeling sick, changes to the menstrual cycle, reduced sexual desire, difficulty reaching sexual orgasm, raised blood pressure, constipation, increased cholesterol. Rare side effects can include an elevated heart rate, severe tremors and increased suicidality.

Drug name: **Mirtazapine**

UK brand names: Zispin

Average doses: 15–30mg per day

What form does it come in? Tablet, orodispersible tablet and liquid

Does it interact with any other medicines? Yes. The following interactions are known:

- *Moclobemide*: Moclobemide and mirtazapine interact badly and should not be taken together
- *Benzodiazepines and sleeping tablets*: Taking mirtazapine alongside medicines that make you drowsy can increase their sedative effects
- *Carbamazepine*: If you take carbamazepine alongside mirtazapine, this can reduce the levels of mirtazapine in your blood, which then makes it less effective

(Continued)

- *Fluoxetine and fluvoxamine*: These two particular SSRIs can interact with mirtazapine and make any side effects more severe
- *MAOI antidepressants*: Serotonin syndrome is more likely if you take mirtazapine alongside an MAOI
- *St John's wort*: You are at an increased risk of developing serotonin syndrome if you take mirtazapine and St John's wort together. St John's wort can also affect the efficacy of mirtazpine

Drug name: Reboxetine

UK brand names: Edronax

Average doses: 4-10mg per day

What form does it come in? Tablet only

Does it interact with any other medicines? Yes. The following interactions are known:

- *MAOI antidepressants*: Serotonin syndrome is more likely if you take reboxetine alongside an MAOI
- *St John's wort*: You are at an increased risk of developing serotonin syndrome if you take reboxetine and St John's wort together. St John's wort can also affect the efficacy of reboxetine

Drug name: Venlafaxine

UK brand names: Effexor, ViePax, Tonpular, Sunveniz, Depefex, Foraven, Politid, Venaxx, Venladex, Venlalic

Average doses: 75-375mg per day

What form does it come in? Tablet and prolonged release capsule

Note: Venlafaxine comes in two forms, regular and XL. If the drug says XL next to it, then this means that the capsule is prolonged release

Does it interact with any other medicines? Yes. The following interactions are known:

- *Antipsychotic medicines (typical)*: Typical antipsychotics interact with venlafaxine and increase the risk of developing a problem with the rhythm of the heart

- *MAOI antidepressants*: Serotonin syndrome is more likely if you take venlafaxine alongside an MAOI
- *Tricyclic antidepressants*: Taking venlafaxine alongside a tricyclic anti-depressant can increase the levels of the tricyclic antidepressant in the blood, and this may lead to increased side effects
- *St John's wort*: You are at an increased risk of developing seroto-nin syndrome if you take venlafaxine and St John's wort together. St John's wort can also affect the efficacy of venlafaxine

ANTIDEPRESSANTS IN PREGNANT WOMEN AND BREASTFEEDING MOTHERS

Managing any medication in pregnancy is difficult, and there needs to be careful consideration of the costs and the benefits of continuing to take the medication compared to stopping the medication, in relation to the health of both mother and baby. If you are working with someone who is pregnant or planning to become pregnant, it is strongly advised that you talk to a specialist practitioner in perinatal mental health before making any decisions around their treatment.

Due to ethical reasons, mental health medicines are not tested on pregnant women, and so the reported risks are only from case study and retrospec-tive reports. This lack of empirical research and clinical trials means that the extent of the impact of antidepressants on unborn babies is not fully known.

If a mother were to come off her antidepressant medication due to preg-nancy or a desire to become pregnant, the key risk would be a possible deterioration in her mood. She would need to have close monitoring and a plan in place in case her mood does start to become low in any way. The risks, to both mother and baby, of the mother developing low mood would need to be considered carefully in each individual case.

In general, the safest type of antidepressant for use in pregnancy is consid-ered to be the tricylclic antidepressants as they carry the lowest risk of causing harm to the baby. However, the risks of tricylic antidepressants remain for the mother, such as side effects, cardiotoxicity and risk of toxicity in overdose.

For all pregnancies, the baby is most vulnerable to harm from medicines in the first three months and in the final month. There is a small but notable risk of premature birth and miscarriage for mothers who are taking any kind of antidepressant medication.

SSRI antidepressants are the type that have been linked with the high-est risk of possible birth defects in the newborn baby, and these defects can include cleft palate, cleft lip, spina bifida and cardiac defects.

If a soon-to-be mother is taking any sort of antidepressant in the final month of her pregnancy, the baby may be at risk of developing withdrawal symptoms from the medication when it is first born. The key withdrawal symptoms to look out for in the baby are:

- *SSRIs and SNRIs*: High blood pressure, low blood sugar, difficulty breathing, crying only very quietly and poor muscle tone.
- *MAOIs and tricyclics*: Muscle spasms, a baby that is 'hard to settle', seizures and a high heart rate.

Specialist perinatal nurses and midwives can support mothers and babies who are in this difficult situation.

All antidepressant medication can be passed to the baby through the breast milk, if the mother chooses to breastfeed, and this may cause the baby to experience side effects similar to the withdrawal symptoms outlined above.

CONSIDERATIONS FOR DIFFERENT AGE GROUPS

Older adults

Antidepressants are safe for use in older adults (age over 65) but falls risk does need to be assessed prior to being prescribed as these medicines can increase both the risk of falls and the risk of injury when a fall occurs. Tricyclic antidepressants in particular should be avoided in older adults due to links with **hypotension**, which increases falls risk. The newer antidepressants such as SSRIs and SNRIs can be used.

Children and young people

Antidepressants are licensed for use for moderate to severe depression in children and young people, but the evidence base is poor and they should always be prescribed by a specialist. Fluoxetine is the only medication currently shown in clinical trials to be effective although it is possible that, in common with the other SSRIs, it is associated with a small increased risk of self-harm and suicidal thoughts (MHRA, 2004).

LEARNING FROM A CASE STUDY: TEST YOUR KNOWLEDGE

Rebecca is a 52-year-old woman who is currently an **informal patient** on an acute psychiatric ward. She has been on the ward for seven weeks and is being treated for an episode of severe depression. Prior to admission, Rebecca tried to end her life by taking an overdose.

Rebecca was first diagnosed with depression after she gave birth to her daughter, an only child, when she was 27 years old, and this is her third admission to hospital. She has taken an overdose of painkillers prior to all of these admissions. During Rebecca's first admission, she was started on an antidepressant tablet called amitriptyline and she took 75mg daily. Rebecca feels that this tablet 'saved her life'.

Rebecca began seeing her GP for feelings of low mood and suicidal thoughts six months ago. These feelings were triggered by a separation from her husband. Rebecca's GP decided to stop her amitriptyline and started her on an antidepressant tablet called sertraline on a dose of 150mg, instead. Since Rebecca changed her medication she feels that her depression has got worse, leading to her overdose and consequent admission.

Rebecca asks to speak to you, as one of the nurses, and she tells you that she thinks that the sertraline tablets that she is taking are 'useless' and so she is not going to take them any more. She says that she does not want to reduce her dose slowly, she just wants to stop taking the tablets altogether:

1   What type of antidepressant is amitriptyline?
2   What type of antidepressant is sertraline?
3   What do you think was behind the GP's decision to switch Rebecca from amitriptyline to sertraline?
4   What might be the risks of Rebecca suddenly stopping her sertraline 150mg?

IF I REMEMBER 5 THINGS FROM THIS CHAPTER...

1   There are four different types of antidepressant medications: tricyclics, MAOIs, SSRIs and SNRIs.
2   Tricylic antidepressants (such as amitriptyline) are highly toxic in overdose. They should not be given to any patient at risk of suicide or of self-harming behaviour.
3   People who take an MAOI antidepressant must avoid consuming a substance called tyramine and so will need to follow a special diet.

(Continued)

4 Serotonin syndrome is a life-threatening condition that can occur in people taking antidepressants when serotonin levels in the brain become too high.
5 Antidepressant medicines should never be stopped suddenly. This can cause the person to feel very unwell and is known as withdrawal syndrome.

ANSWERS TO THE CASE STUDY QUESTIONS

1 Amitriptyline is a tricyclic antidepressant.
2 Sertraline is an SSRI antidepressant.
3 The GP may have been concerned about the risk of Rebecca taking a fatal overdose of her amitriptyline. Amitriptyline is highly toxic in overdose, and so should not be prescribed for individuals who are feeling suicidal. Rebecca was expressing thoughts of ending her life and also has a history of taking overdoses, which increases the likelihood of this potential risk.
4 If Rebecca suddenly stops taking her sertraline, she is at risk of withdrawal syndrome. This may increase Rebecca's feelings of suicidality and may also cause her depression to become even more severe. Physically, Rebecca may feel like she has flu and feel dizzy. Her sleep may become affected, and she may have increased feelings of anxiety and irritability.

REFERENCES AND RECOMMENDED READING

Gott, M., Hinchliff, S. and Galena, E. (2004) 'General practitioner attitudes towards discussing sexual health issues with older people', *Social Science and Medicine*, 58: 2003–13.

Jiaquan Xu, M.D., Sherry, L., Murphy, B.S., et al. (2016) 'Deaths: Final data for 2013', *National Vital Statistics Reports*, 64 (2): 1–119.

Kotliar, D.M. (2016) 'Depression narratives in blogs: A collaborative question for coherence', *Qualitative Health Research*, 26 (9): 1203–15.

Kring, A.M., Davison, G.C. and Neale, J.M. (2013) *Abnormal Psychology*. London: John Wiley and Sons.

Mind (2020) 'Antidepressants A–Z.' Available at: www.mind.org.uk/information-support/drugs-and-treatments/antidepressants-a-z/overview (accessed 25 June 2021).

MHRA (2014) Selective serotonin reuptake inhibitors (SSRIs) and serotonin and noradrenaline reuptake inhibitors (SNRIs): use and safety. Available at: www.gov.uk/government/publications/ssris-and-snris-use-and-safety/ selective-serotonin-reuptake-inhibitors-ssris-and-serotonin-and-noradrenaline-reuptake-inhibitors-snris-use-and-safety (accessed 4th November 2021).

Moncrieff, J. (2011) 'Questioning the neuroprotective hypothesis: Does drug treatment prevent brain damage in early psychosis or schizophrenia?', *British Journal of Psychiatry*, 198 (2): 85–7.

NICE (2016) 'First-choice antidepressant use in adults with depression or generalised anxiety disorder.' Available at: www.nice.org.uk/advice/ktt8/chapter/Evidence-context (accessed 24 June 2021).

Nursing and Midwifery Council (NMC) (2020) The Code. Available at: www.nmc.org.uk/standards/code (accessed 25 June 2021).

Office for National Statistics (ONS) (2021) 'Coronavirus and depression in adults, Great Britain: January to March 2021.' Available at: www.ons.gov.uk/peoplepopulationandcommunity/wellbeing/articles/coronavirusanddepressioninadultsgreatbritain/januarytomarch2021 (accessed 25 June 2021).

Rottmann, L.H. (1986) 'Depression: The common cold of mental health', *Extension Circular*, 86–416.

Royal College of Psychiatrists (2014) 'Coming off anti-depressants'. Available at: www.rcpsych.ac.uk/healthadvice/treatmentswellbeing/antidepressants/comingoffantidepressants.aspx (accessed 22 August 2016).

Uher, R., Farmer, A., Henigsberg, N., et al. on behalf of the Royal College of Psychiatrists (2009) 'Adverse reactions to anti-depressants', *British Journal of Psychiatry*, 195 (3): 202–10.

2 MOOD-STABILISING MEDICATIONS

LIZ HOLLAND

AFTER READING THIS CHAPTER, YOU WILL BE ABLE TO:

- Discuss what we mean by the term 'bipolar disorder' and understand what a person with bipolar disorder may experience
- Discuss the five most commonly prescribed medicines that are used to help stabilise mood
- Define the term '**polypharmacy**' and relate this to bipolar disorder
- Be aware of the monitoring requirements for the drug lithium
- Understand the risks of lithium toxicity
- Discuss the complexities of prescribing mood-stabilising medicines for women of childbearing age
- Apply this knowledge to a clinical scenario

WHEN MIGHT MOOD-STABILISING MEDICATIONS BE USED?

The use of mood-stabilising medication is seen when someone is being treated for 'bipolar disorder'.

Bipolar disorder is a mood disorder characterised by extreme fluctuations in mood. A person with bipolar disorder will have periods of very low mood and low energy (depressive episodes) and periods of very high mood and high energy (manic episodes). The person may also have periods of time where they seem excitable and elated but are not as high as when they are in a full manic episode; this is known as 'hypomania'.

There are three known categories of bipolar disorder. Bipolar 1 is characterised by both depressive episodes and manic episodes and can lead to the person needing hospital care very quickly, as the manic episodes can be quite extreme. A person with bipolar 2 also has depressive episodes, but the episodes of elated mood only ever reach the hypomanic threshold. 'Cyclothymia' (bipolar 3) is the mildest form of bipolar disorder, where the person will have periods of both high and low mood but will not reach the levels of a full depressive or hypomanic episode.

When people are going through an episode of mania their behaviour can become erratic and bizarre: they may say and do things that they would not normally say and do, and behave in ways that they would not normally behave. When people are manic they may also develop symptoms of psychosis. Manic episodes are the time in which people with bipolar disorder are most likely to need the support of hospital admission and care (National Institute of Mental Health, 2016):

> I began to believe that my step father was behind why I was in hospital and wouldn't let him see me, I thought that the doctors and nurses were a gang holding me hostage. I was fearful of everything, talking and singing to myself, unable to sit still and became quite agitated at times with the staff and patients, which is completely out of character for me. I simply didn't know what was real or unreal and I was so frightened of the staff and others while my brain was in this state.
>
> (In a blog for the Time to Change campaign, 2017, Sarah details her experience of having a psychotic episode whilst going through a period of mania)

Bipolar disorder can respond very well to medicines, but often more than one medicine is used in order to help the person. The term that we use when people take more than one medicine is 'polypharmacy'. The person will often take an antidepressant medicine that will help with their tendency to low mood, and a mood-stabilising medicine that will help their mood to remain stable. The use of antidepressant medications in people with bipolar disorder needs to be managed very carefully, as taking too much of an antidepressant medication can cause someone to become elated in their mood and consequently develop a manic episode. When the person is going through a manic episode they may take some extra medication (such as a benzodiazepine) in order to quickly help them feel calmer. A person may also take some short-term medicine to help them with their sleep when they are having a severe depressive or manic episode, as both of these can have a notable impact on sleeping patterns. If the person develops signs and symptoms of psychosis whilst in a manic episode, an antipsychotic medicine may be used in order to help.

This chapter will discuss the use of mood-stabilising medications as information on antidepressant medications is covered in Chapter 1, and information on medicines that can quickly calm someone down is covered in both Chapter 3 and Chapter 6. Information on medicines that help with sleep is covered in Chapter 3. Information on antipsychotic medications is discussed in Chapter 5.

WHICH MEDICATIONS ARE USED TO HELP STABILISE MOOD?

There are five key medications that are often used in practice as mood-stabilising medications in the UK. These are:

- Lithium
- Valproate
- Carbamazepine
- Lamotrigine
- Asenapine.

The current NICE guidelines (2015) for management of bipolar disorder state that choosing what to prescribe is bespoke to each individual and should be informed by other medications the person is taking and any known previous responses to medications. The NICE (2020) update specifies that any person being treated with lithium or valproate should be under a specialist secondary mental health service before starting this medication.

The Independent Medicines and Medical Devices Safety Review (IMMDS, 2020) notes the risks of valproate, and this has led to the development of a national "Valporate Safety Implementation Group" hosted by NHS England, which is coordinating work that aims, by 2023, to reduce by 50 per cent the use of valproate in people who can get pregnant, and to help prevent unplanned pregnancies in this group of patients. You can read more about the group and the actions they are taking at: www.england.nhs.uk/patient-safety/sodium-valproate

---

GO FURTHER ...

If you would like to read more about how different medicines prescribed for mood stabilisation compare with each other, a good read to start you off is an article by Keck and McElroy (2002).

These are not all from the same family of medicines. Lithium is a natural mineral, rather than a drug that is artificially developed by the pharmaceutical industry. Asenapine is an antipsychotic by nature but is not used for the treatment of psychosis at present; it is only used for mood stabilisation. As it is a very new drug, there is still not much information or evidence behind it. Valproate, lamotrigine and carbamazepine are all anticonvulsant medications. This means that they are often prescribed for the management of epilepsy and seizures, but they have also been found to have mood-stabilising properties.

GO FURTHER ...

If you would like to read more about how anticonvulsant medications work, then the article by Stahl (2004) is recommended.

Choosing which mood-stabilising medicine is right for someone is a difficult decision to make, as they all have their own side effects, and these can be severe. In general, lithium is found to be particularly effective in people who have bipolar 1. Asenapine is only likely to be prescribed if other mood stabilisers have been found to be ineffective. Carbamazepine or valproate can be a good choice for people who move quickly between periods of high mood and low mood. Lamotrigine is more likely to be used in bipolar 2 than bipolar 1.

Of all of these medications, lithium has the most complex side effect profile, and is subject to special monitoring requirements.

LITHIUM MONITORING

Due to the risks and side effects associated with lithium, special monitoring processes are required. When a person is commenced on lithium, they will be assigned a lithium treatment pack in order to help keep this monitoring process on track, and to provide a clear record of the monitoring. This pack is in purple, and all the information associated with lithium monitoring will also be in purple. The pack includes a booklet in which all blood test results can be recorded, a Lithium Alert Card for the person to keep with them that will indicate that they are taking lithium, and a lithium therapy information booklet. Some organisations/NHS trusts will also have their own booklets or monitoring documents that need to be completed, so do check what your organisations are using.

The Lithium Alert Card can be seen in Figure 2.1.

Lithium Alert Card

This patient is taking lithium therapy
This card should be carried at all times and shown to healthcare professionals

Name of patent:

Address:

Postcode: Telephone:

GP:

NHS number: _ _ _   _ _ _   _ _ _ _

Figure 2.1   Lithium Alert Card

All patients taking lithium will need to have regular blood tests in order to assess their lithium level, which is the measure of how much lithium there is in their blood. The safe range for the lithium level is 0.4–1.0mmol/L.

The factors that influence a person's lithium level are varied, but include metabolic rate, weight, salt intake, exercise levels and fluid consumption. A person's dose of lithium will be adjusted until their lithium level falls to within the safe range of 0.4–1.0mmol/L. Once a person's lithium dose is stable, the person will be asked not to adjust any lifestyle factors that could affect their fluid balance, such as fluid consumption and salt intake.

All blood tests for lithium levels should be taken around 12 hours after a person has taken their dose of lithium. When a person is starting on lithium treatment or has undergone a dose change, the person should have their lithium level taken weekly until the bloods are returning stable results. The person should then go to three-monthly monitoring. If the person has any lifestyle changes that may affect sodium and fluid levels, they will need to go back to weekly monitoring until their blood levels are stable.

In addition to the above blood monitoring, the person will need additional health monitoring. Prior to anyone starting on lithium, their baseline renal, cardiac and thyroid function will need to be tested, and then renal, cardiac and thyroid function should be assessed every six months.

LITHIUM TOXICITY

When a person's blood lithium level goes *higher than 1.5mmol/L*, the person is at risk of lithium toxicity. Lithium toxicity can occur at any time in a person taking lithium. Any concerns about lithium toxicity must be acted upon quickly, because if it is not treated promptly, it can be fatal.

Lithium toxicity will present with some key symptoms. These are:

- Blurred vision
- Dizziness
- Difficulty walking
- Slurred speech
- Muscle twitches in the arms and legs
- Trembling hands and legs
- Vomiting or severe nausea
- Persistent diarrhoea
- Swollen feet and/or legs
- An irregular heartbeat
- A rash.

If a person who is taking lithium presents with any of the above symptoms, they should be closely monitored, and their blood should be taken in order to obtain a lithium level immediately. They should not be given their next dose of lithium until their blood results come back and are normal. These should be processed as 'urgent'.

SUPPORTING THE TREATMENT OF BIPOLAR WITH ANTIPSYCHOTIC MEDICATIONS

As mentioned above, we are increasingly seeing people who live with bipolar disorder taking antipsychotic medication as part of their treatment plans. Prescribing an antipsychotic medication needs careful consideration of risks and benefits, in particular around the risks of physical health complications and weight gain (see Chapter 6).

Antipsychotic medication is often used for those who are experiencing a manic episode, as it can be helpful with agitation, distress and difficulty sleeping, hallucinations or delusions that the person is currently experiencing. The use of antipsychotics can also impact on how other medications are working. The medications we tend to see being used most often are olanzapine and quetiapine. Please see Chapter 6 for more information on these medications, side effects and monitoring.

THE MEDICINES LIST

This medicines list will provide information on the five key mood-stabilising medicines that are used in the UK, as outlined above. This is not an exhaustive list of all the possible treatments that can be used for the treatment of bipolar.

Drug name: **Lithium**

UK brand names: Camcolit, Liskonum, Lithonate, Priadel, Litarex, Li-Liquid

Average doses: Depends on the individual patient and is determined by regularly monitoring the lithium level in the blood. An average starting dose on lithium tablets may be around 400mg a day. The person's age and weight should also be considered when lithium is being prescribed

What form does it come in? Liquid and tablet

Does it interact with any other medications? Yes. The following interactions are known:

- *Lithium should not be taken with*: Antibiotic medications or steroid medications without medical advice, medicines containing caffeine, water tablets, creams containing urea, non-steroidal anti-inflammatory (NSAID) **analgesic** medications (such as ibuprofen). Medical advice should be obtained for anyone on blood pressure or cardiac medication if they are also prescribed lithium

Additional information: See the section above on lithium monitoring. Lithium should not be taken by anyone with severe kidney or thyroid difficulties. Lithium can cause an itchy rash in some people. If this occurs, it should be stopped immediately and medical advice should be sought

---

Anticonvulsant medications

In rare cases, these medicines can be associated with an increased risk of suicidal thoughts. People taking these medicines should also keep an eye out for any skin rashes and serious flu-like symptoms, as these can be warning signs of Stevens–Johnson syndrome, which can be fatal.

Drug name: Valproate

UK brand names: Epilim, Depakote

Average doses: Usually, between 1000 and 2000mg per day

What form does it come in? Liquid and tablet

Does it interact with any other medicines? Yes. The following interactions are known:

- *Other medicines*: Medical advice must be sought if valproate is being taken with salicylate painkillers (e.g. aspirin), other medicines for epilepsy, blood-thinning medications, medicines to reduce cholesterol, medicines for HIV, medicines for cancer, antidepressant medications, antipsychotic medications
- *MAOI antidepressants*: Valproate must not be taken with MAOI antidepressants

Additional information: Valproate should not be taken by anyone with liver problems

Drug name: Carbamazepine

UK brand names: Carbagen SR, Tegretol, Tegretol Retard, Teril Retard

Average doses: Usually, up to 1200mg per day

What form does it come in? Liquid and tablet

Does it interact with any other medicines? Yes. The following interactions are known:

- *MAOI antidepressants*: Carbamazepine must not be taken with any MAOI antidepressants
- *St John's wort*: Carbamazepine must not be taken with St John's wort

(Continued)

- *Other medicines*: Medical advice must be sought before starting carbamazepine if a person is taking other medicines for epilepsy, anticoagulants, omeprazole, any antipsychotic medication, any antidepressant medication, any medicine used to treat sickness, antibiotics, water tablets, hormone replacement therapy (HRT), antifungals, corticosteroids, painkillers, asthma medicines, oral contraceptives (as efficacy of these can be decreased), levothyroxine, medicines for cancer, medicines for HIV, bupropion, antihistamines, vitamin B supplements

Additional information: MAOI antidepressants must have been stopped at least two weeks prior to starting carbamazepine. Carbamazepine should not be taken by anyone with a heart condition. The patient on carbamazepine must not drink alcohol or eat/drink grapefruit

Drug name: **Lamotrigine**

UK brand names: Lamictal

Average doses: Usually, 100–400mg per day

What form does it come in? Tablet and dispersible tablet

Does it interact with any other medicines? Yes. The following interactions are known:

- *Other medicines*: Medical advice must be sought if lamotrigine is being taken with any other medicines for epilepsy, olanzapine, risperidone, lithium, aripiprazole, carbamazepine, bupropion, rifampicin, medicines for HIV, oral contraceptives

Additional information: Caution should be taken for people with kidney problems

Asenapine

Asenapine is a second-generation antipsychotic. A key side effect of asenapine is that it can initially cause low blood pressure. This may cause some people to feel dizzy or to faint when they move or stand up suddenly. Asenapine is also associated with involuntary rhythmic movements of the tongue, mouth and face, and it carries a risk of neuroleptic malignant syndrome (NMS). You can read more about NMS in Chapter 5.

Drug name: **Asenapine**

UK brand names: Sycrest

Average doses: One 5mg or 10mg tablet, twice per day. Usual daily maximum is 20mg.

What form does it come in? 5mg and 10mg sublingual tablets (these should be placed under the tongue until they dissolve)

Does it interact with any other medications: Yes. The following interactions are known:

- *Antidepressant*: Asenapine can interact with antidepressant medication (in particular, fluvoxamine, fluoxetine or paroxetine)
- *Medicines for Parkinson's disease*: These can make asenapine less effective
- *Medicines that lower blood pressure*: Asenapine should not be taken with any other medicines that lower blood pressure

Additional information: Asenapine should not be used in older adults (usually over 60). People with liver problems should not take asenapine. You should not drink alcohol when taking asenapine. You must not eat or drink for at least ten minutes after taking a dose of asenapine. If you are taking more than one medicine, asenapine should always be taken last

MEDICINES FOR MOOD STABILISATION IN PREGNANT WOMEN AND BREASTFEEDING MOTHERS

It should be noted that all of the mood-stabilising medications carry risks in relation to unborn children, and for pregnant women taking mood stabilisers there is currently no preferred option. Any women who are pregnant or planning on becoming pregnant and who are taking a mood-stabilising medication will need to work with a specialist in order to plan the safest possible treatment for both them and their baby.

The highest risk types of mood-stabilising medication for unborn babies are the anticonvulsant medications. Taking an anticonvulsant when pregnant can lead to 'fetal anticonvulsant syndrome', which can cause both physical and cognitive defects in the baby and is associated with developmental delay. The first three months of pregnancy is the highest-risk time for this.

Valproate carries the highest potential risks of all the anticonvulsant medications. It is best practice to avoid prescribing valproate to any woman of childbearing age due to the potential risks to the baby if she were to get pregnant. If valproate is seen as the best treatment choice, then the clinician and the woman would need to discuss if and when she would like to get pregnant, and her current use of contraception. Specific risks of valproate in relation to the unborn baby include an increased risk of spina bifida and other spinal abnormalities, cleft palate and cleft lip abnormalities, heart defects, abnormal fingers and toes, extra fingers and toes and an increased risk of the baby being born with an intellectual disability.

Anticonvulsant medicines are much less risky once the baby is born, and the risks associated with breastfeeding and taking such medicines are low.

As asenapine is such a new drug, there is currently very little research available, and knowledge about its use in pregnant and breastfeeding mothers is limited.

Taking lithium during pregnancy carries noted risks both to the mother and to the unborn child, and very careful monitoring of both mother and baby is required if it is decided that continuing with lithium treatment is the best course of action. In relation to the baby, the most well-known risk is that of heart defects if lithium is taken during early pregnancy. There is also an increased risk of a baby being stillborn or of sudden death after the baby is born. As discussed above, careful fluid balancing is always important to anyone taking lithium, and this is particularly important if a woman is pregnant. During pregnancy, liver and kidney function change, as do fluid and hormone levels, meaning that a woman's lithium level can change rapidly during pregnancy. Extra lithium-level monitoring is therefore required for pregnant women. Childbirth itself is also a high-risk time for pregnant women taking lithium due to both the sudden changes in fluid balance and to the fact that the way in which the body metabolises lithium changes in labour.

Women taking lithium are advised not to breastfeed as lithium is passed through the breast milk from mother to baby and can lead to the baby having harmful lithium levels in their blood.

CONSIDERATIONS FOR DIFFERENT AGE GROUPS

The peak age of onset for bipolar disorder is in late adolescence or early adult life, with a further small increase in incidence in mid to late life (NICE, 2015). Diagnosis and treatment of any possible bipolar disorder in a child should be undertaken by a specialist service as the diagnostic criteria are not tailored to young people, and consequent treatment will be bespoke.

For those over 65, treatment by someone who specialises in working with older adults is recommended. The NICE guidelines state that approaches to treatment will be the same, but doses may need to be lower and to be calculated with age in mind. The falls risks associated with sedating medications must also be considered. NICE (2020) states that for medications given to older adults, the following considerations must be applied:

- use medication at lower doses
- take into account the increased risk of drug interactions
- take into account the negative impact that anticholinergic medication, or drugs with anticholinergic activity, can have on cognitive function and mobility
- ensure that medical comorbidities have been recognised and treated.

LEARNING FROM A CASE STUDY: TEST YOUR KNOWLEDGE

Dana is 31 years old and was diagnosed with bipolar disorder at the age of 19. Dana takes the mood-stabilising drug lithium in tablet form, which works really well for her. She has not had a hospital admission in over three years. Dana has a lithium information pack at home and carries her Lithium Alert Card in her purse. She has been taking the same dose of lithium for the last three years and manages her fluid and salt intake to ensure that this remains stable.

1   What colour is Dana's information pack and card?

Dana has been dating a new partner, Delroy, for almost a year, and things are getting serious. They have just decided to move in together, and hope for a future that involves marriage and children. Delroy asks her for more information about her lithium treatment so that he can support her. He would like to know about what monitoring she requires and if there are any risks.

(Continued)

2   How often does Dana need to have her lithium bloods taken, and what is the safe range for her lithium blood levels?
3   Does Dana need any other regular health checks?
4   If Dana and Delroy decide to try for a baby, does Dana need to think about anything concerning her medications before she stops taking her contraceptive pill?

One day, Dana comes home from work early as she has not been feeling well. She feels sick and has had diarrhoea for the last few days. When Delroy comes home from work, he notices that Dana does not seem her usual self. Her speech is slurred, and she seems wobbly on her feet. He notices that her hands are shaking. Dana tells Delroy that she feels dizzy and her heart is pounding. Delroy gets cross with Dana and starts shouting at her, telling her that she is clearly drunk.

5   Is there another explanation that may be causing Dana's symptoms? What should Delroy do?

IF I REMEMBER 5 THINGS FROM THIS CHAPTER...

1   There are five commonly used mood-stabilising medicines used in the UK. These are: lithium, carbamazepine, valproate, lamotrigine and asenapine.
2   There are considerable risks when any mood-stabilising medicine is taken by a pregnant woman, and the fetus is at risk of harm. Valproate carries the highest risk to the baby. Specialist advice must be sought if a woman who takes a mood-stabilising medicine becomes pregnant or wishes to become pregnant.
3   Anyone who takes lithium will have a purple lithium information pack.
4   Anyone who takes lithium must have regular blood monitoring tests; the safe lithium blood level is: 0.4-1.0mmol/L.
5   Lithium toxicity occurs when a person's lithium level is over 1.5 mmol/L. It can occur to anyone at any time, and symptoms must be looked out for at all times because if it is not treated early it can be fatal.

ANSWERS TO THE CASE STUDY QUESTIONS

1   Purple.
2   Dana should be having her lithium levels checked every three months, and the safe range is 0.4-1.0 mmol/L.

3   In addition, Dana should be having her renal, cardiac and thyroid function checked every six months.
4   Yes. Dana needs to meet with her doctor before she comes off her contraceptive pill in order to obtain some advice. If she continues on her lithium and becomes pregnant then there are risks to both her and her baby, and so additional monitoring will need to be arranged for them both.
5   These could also be signs that Dana's lithium level is becoming toxic. Delroy should take Dana to A&E immediately, and he should also take her lithium information pack, blood test record book and Alert Card with him. He should explain that Dana is on lithium and that he is very worried that she is becoming toxic because of the symptoms that she is demonstrating. He should clearly describe these symptoms. He should take Dana's lithium tablets with them to A&E.

REFERENCES AND RECOMMENDED READING

British National Formulary (BNF) and National Institute for Health and Care Excellence (NICE) (2017) 'Lithium carbonate monitoring requirements'. Available at: https://bnf.nice.org.uk/drug/lithium-carbonate. html#monitoringRequirements (accessed 25 June 2017).

IMMDS (2020) *First Do No Harm: The Report of the Independent Medicines and Medical Devices Safety Review*. Available at https://immdsreview.org.uk/downloads/IMMDSReview_Web.pdf (accessed 30 June 2021).

Keck, P.E and McElroy, S.E. (2002) 'Antiepileptic drugs for bipolar disorder: Are there any clear winners?', *Current Psychiatry*, 1 (1): 18–24.

Mind (2015) 'Lithium and other mood stabilisers'. Available at: https://mind.org.uk/information-support/drugs-and-treatments/lithium-and-other-mood-stabilisers/#.WU-_rjBTFyQ (accessed 25 June 2017).

National Institute of Mental Health (NIMH) (2016) 'Bipolar disorder'. Available at: www.nimh.nih.gov/health/topics/bipolar-disorder/index.shtml (accessed 25 June 2017).

NHS England (2021) 'Sodium valporate'. Available at www.england.nhs.uk/patient-safety/sodium-valproate (accessed 28 June 2021).

NICE (2015) 'Bipolar disorder: The management of bipolar disorder in adults, children and adolescents, in primary and secondary care'. Available at: www.nice.org.uk/guidance/cg38/documents/bipolar-disorder-first-consultation-nice-guideline2 (accessed 28 June 2021).

NICE (2020) 'Bipolar disorder: Assessment and management'. Available at www.nice.org.uk/guidance/cg185/chapter/1-recommendations#how-to-use-medication (accessed 28 June 2021).

Package information leaflet for asenapine tablets (2017) Available at: www.medicines.org.uk/emc/PIL.25633.latest.pdf (accessed 25 June 2017).

Package information leaflet for Tegretol (carbamazepine) tablets (2021) Available at: www.medicines.org.uk/emc/medicine/4095#gref (accessed 4 November 2021).

Package information leaflet for lamotrigine tablets (2017) Available at: www.medicines.org.uk/emc/PIL.25854.latest.pdf (accessed 25 June 2017).

Package information leaflet for lithium carbonate tablets – Lithium Carbonate Essential Pharma 250 mg film-coated tablets (2021) Available at: www.medicines.org.uk/emc/product/10828/smpc (accessed 4 November 2021).

Package information leaflet for sodium valproate tablets (2017) Available at: www.medicines.org.uk/emc/PIL.32982.latest.pdf (accessed 25 June 2017).

Stahl, S.M. (2004) 'Psychopharmacology of anti-convulsants: Do all anti-convulsants have the same mechanism of action?', *Journal of Clinical Psychiatry*, 65 (2): 149–50.

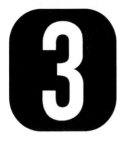

3 MEDICATIONS FOR MANAGING ANXIETY INCLUDING COMMON SLEEP MEDICATIONS

LIZ HOLLAND

AFTER READING THIS CHAPTER, YOU WILL BE ABLE TO:

- Describe what we mean by 'anxiety' and 'panic'
- Have an understanding of the treatment options for people suffering from acute anxiety and from anxiety disorders
- List the different categories of medicines used to treat anxiety and be able to give examples
- Apply this knowledge to a clinical scenario

WHEN DO WE NEED TO USE MEDICATIONS FOR MANAGING ANXIETY?

'Anxiety' refers to the way we feel when we are facing a difficult, challenging or threatening situation. For many people, transient and temporary feelings of anxiety are a normal part of life and do not present a difficulty. However, at least one in ten of us has issues with feelings of anxiety which become problematic, often known as 'anxiety disorders' (Royal College of Psychiatrists, 2014).

With anxiety disorders, there are both psychological and physical symptoms that the person will experience during an episode of anxiety. In terms of psychological symptoms, the person will have worries constantly going through their mind, feel very tired, grumpy or irritable, find it hard to concentrate on things and have difficulties sleeping. In terms of the physical symptoms, the person may have achy muscles, tensions and pains, a racing heartbeat, feel sweaty, have heavy shallow breathing, feel shaky or visibly shake, feel faint, feel dizzy and have gastrointestinal disturbances such as feeling sick, having diarrhoea or indigestion. For people with anxiety disorders, these feelings can come on suddenly with no apparent trigger. This can be incredibly distressing.

For some people with anxiety disorders, these feelings of anxiety can develop into a full-blown panic attack. This is a very scary experience for the person. When someone has a panic attack they will feel a sense of impending doom and often that they are about to die. The person will feel that their heart is pounding and beating irregularly, and they will take rapid, shallow breaths. They will often appear sweaty and disorientated:

> It came upon me by surprise. I began to feel wave after wave of fear and my stomach gave out on me. I could hear my heart pounding so loudly I thought it would come out of my chest. Pains were shooting down my legs. I became so afraid I couldn't catch my breath. What was happening to me? Was I having a heart attack? Was I dying? (Richards, 2016)

Often with anxiety and panic, the most effective treatments are psychological interventions such as cognitive behavioural therapy (CBT). These help the person to find the roots of their feelings of panic and anxiety, and also to manage their thoughts, identify warning signs of anxiety and panic, and develop techniques to help them manage the psychological and physical symptoms.

GO FURTHER ...

'Mindfulness' is a psychological intervention that is becoming more popular and can be really powerful in helping to relieve feelings of anxiety, panic, stress and low mood. It refers to how a person can focus on themselves and ground themselves in the moment. You can read a simple description at www.nhs.uk/Conditions/stress-anxiety-depression/Pages/mindfulness.aspx, and follow a link to the NICE guidelines on mindfulness.

If you would like to start reading in more depth around mindfulness, begin with Groves (2016). There is a link to the article in the References at the end of this chapter.

Coping strategies and distraction can also be a very useful tool in supporting the onset of sudden panic. Psychological interventions for anxiety focus on helping the person to separate the anxiety into thoughts, feelings, physiological sensations and behaviours. The idea is that the person is supported to identify their own early warning signs of anxiety – for many people this may start with a difficult or negative thought, but for others, especially those with lived experience of trauma, it may well be a physiological sensation such as butterflies in the stomach or suddenly feeling hot and sweaty. It is really helpful to talk with those you are supporting about how anxiety comes on for them, and identify these early indicators. You can then work with the person to try out different coping and distraction techniques to see what helps to stop the anxiety from continuing to take hold. One coping technique that many people find helpful is 'square breathing'. With this, you take a deep breath in over four seconds, hold the breath for four seconds, breathe out over four seconds, hold your breath for four seconds and repeat.

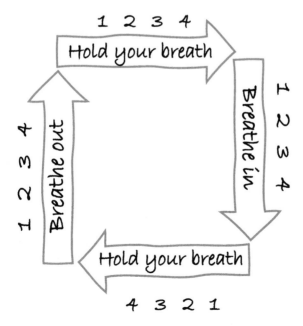

Figure 3.1 Square breathing

Another good exercise that is fun to try (assuming the person does not have any health needs like diabetes or swallowing or choking issues) is to place a very sour sweet or piece of chocolate on the end of the tongue, close your eyes and focus on the taste and the sensation, which can be very grounding.

In cases of severe anxiety, medication may be prescribed. This will often be a short-term solution in order to help the person whilst they are in crisis, and the person will usually undertake some sort of psychological treatment alongside the pharmacological treatment, with the aim being to help them reduce their use of medication once they have completed the psychological interventions.

WHAT ARE THE DIFFERENT TYPES OF MEDICATIONS FOR MANAGING ANXIETY AND HOW DO THEY WORK?

There are three main categories of medication that are commonly used as pharmacological interventions for anxiety. These are: *tranquillisers, antidepressants* and *beta blockers*. There is also an anticonvulsant medication known as pregabalin, which is licensed for use in anxiety. Each has a different effect and works differently. Each will now be discussed in more depth. In practice, you may see rare occasions in which very low-dose antipsychotics are prescribed for the management of anxiety. However, this is highly specialist so it will not be discussed further in this chapter.

Tranquillisers

These are the medicines often referred to as 'anti-anxiety' drugs, due to their direct impact on the reduction of symptoms of anxiety. They work by slowing down the central nervous system reactions, consequently reducing brain activity and helping to induce a sense of calm. As they reduce the feelings of anxiety, they can also make the person feel sleepy; hence, many tranquillisers are also prescribed as sleeping aids.

Barbiturates and benzodiazepines are the most well-known categories of medication for anxiety. Barbiturates were the most commonly used until the start of the 1960s; however, at the time it was noted that they were highly addictive as well as having very unpleasant side effects, and benzodiazepines became the more popular choice from this point.

Barbiturates and benzodiazepines work in a similar way by stimulating the production of a neurotransmitter known as gamma-aminobutyric acid (GABA), and GABA is linked to feelings of calm.

Benzodiazepines (e.g. clonazepam, temazepam, lorazepam, diazepam) are noted for their addictive properties, and it should also be noted that people very quickly develop a tolerance to benzodiazepines, meaning that increasingly high doses have to be prescribed over time. Hence, it is recommended that any treatment with benzodiazepines should be short term, ideally no longer than four weeks. In general, benzodiazepines should not be given to people who are aged 60 years or older as, in this age group, the drugs can increase disorientation and risk of falling and cause the person to become more agitated rather than less.

There are two different types of benzodiazepines: short acting and long acting. The short-acting medicines, such as lorazepam, are often given as 'PRN' (as required) medication and are discussed in further detail in Chapter 6. There are also long-acting medications, such as clonazepam, which may be used for maintenance treatment rather than for a crisis situation. People with severe anxiety disorders are likely to be prescribed a short-term regimen of long-acting benzodiazepines but may also have short-acting medicines available for additional use when they are having a sudden moment of crisis. If someone is taking a regular dose of a long-acting benzodiazepine, it is often recommended that this medicine is taken at night due to the associated feelings of drowsiness.

Once someone is taking a regular dose of a benzodiazepine, it is important that they do not suddenly stop taking the medication as this can lead to withdrawal effects, which can range from headaches, tremors, sleep disturbances, confusion, feeling sick and muscular pain to having seizures and hallucinations. It is recommended that the person is gradually withdrawn from the medication by slowly decreasing the dose over a period of weeks.

Another type of tranquilliser often used in the treatment of anxiety is sleeping medication. This is because people who have problems with anxiety and panic often have difficulty sleeping. The most commonly prescribed sleeping drug is zopiclone, followed by zolpidem. These are modern sleeping medicines and are known as the 'z' medications for sleep. They also work by stimulating GABA production, but have been found to be less addictive. They are fast acting and so should be taken by the person when they are approaching their bedtime. They can sometimes leave the person feeling drowsy and 'hung over' when they wake up in the morning, and so it is important to ensure awareness of this; for example, you would not want someone to wake up after using a sleeping medication and then have to drive a car. NICE guidelines for use of these medications (2019) state that if a person has tried a 'z' medication for sleep and it has not been helpful, another 'z' medication should not be tried instead. They also state that their use must be closely monitored, and they must only be prescribed for controlled periods.

Antidepressant

There is a growing body of evidence that antidepressant medications can be effective in helping to reduce the symptoms of extreme anxiety and panic. Anxiety disorders and depression are often comorbid; this means that people will often have a diagnosis of both an anxiety disorder and depression. Antidepressant medications tend to be used as a more long-term treatment than benzodiazepines, which are short term. The SSRI family of antidepressants tend to be the most effective in the treatment of anxiety and panic. You can read more about SSRIs in Chapter 1.

Antidepressant medication can take up to about six weeks to be effective, and so you may need to use a short-term benzodiazepine whilst getting the person started on an antidepressant, which may be the longer-term treatment.

Some of the most commonly prescribed antidepressants for anxiety include fluoxetine, sertraline, citalopram and paroxetine.

Beta blockers

Beta blockers (propranolol, atenolol) may be prescribed as an initial intervention, or be prescribed alongside other medications in the treatment of anxiety. They are effective in reducing the physical symptoms of anxiety and panic but do not address the root causes of anxiety. They can help reduce a rapid heart rate, a pounding heart and shakiness, and they work by blocking the action of the neurotransmitter, norepinephrine. Beta blockers are not addictive but they can impact on your blood pressure, which is why you should not suddenly stop taking them. They are usually used on prescription for helping to reduce blood pressure in people with hypertension; hence, low blood pressure can be one of the side effects. Other side effects include a slow heart rate, cold hands and feet, sickness and diarrhoea, dizziness, tiredness and blurred vision.

Pregabalin and buspirone

Pregabalin is an anticonvulsant medication that is typically used to treat epilepsy. However, it has been noted to have beneficial uses in the reduction of feelings of anxiety and panic, and can be used for long-term treatment. A benefit of pregabalin is that it has a better side effect profile than antidepressants, which is the other option for longer-term treatment; pregabalin does not typically have gastrointestinal (GI) complications such as nausea and also does not tend to cause sexual side effects such as vaginal dryness or difficulties in gaining an erection. Pregabalin is, however, linked with increased appetite and weight gain, headache, dry mouth, feelings of **vertigo**, dizziness, drowsiness and blurred vision. The precise way in which pregabalin works to reduce anxiety is still unclear; however, it is thought that it is in part due to its impact on calcium channels within the brain, and its impact on the neurotransmitter, norepinephrine. An older medication similar to pregabalin which you may also come into contact with is gabapentin.

Buspirone is specifically known as an anti-anxiety medication (anxiolytic) and has been around for about 30 years. It can be a good medication to use in those susceptible to side effects, as the side effect profile is quite low, and in particular it does not have sexual side effects. Buspirone can also be a good choice for those where there is a risk of accidental or non-accidental overdose.

WHAT IMPORTANT INFORMATION DO I NEED TO DISCUSS WITH PEOPLE TAKING BENZODIAZEPINE MEDICATIONS FOR ANXIETY?

It is really important that from the moment the person starts taking a benzodiazepine you explain clearly that it is a short-term-only treatment, and you also need to ensure that a referral for psychological interventions has been made. Make sure that the person is aware of the possible symptoms of **addiction** so that they can keep an eye out for these and ask for help. These include:

- Craving the next dose
- Becoming more tolerant to the drugs being taken
- Feeling tense and agitated
- Feeling guilty if you miss a dose
- Struggling to sleep
- Feeling dizzy.

You should also advise anyone taking a new medication of the side effects that they may experience, and for benzodiazepines, the most common include:

- Feeling confused
- Feeling drowsy and sleepy
- Feeling dizzy
- Slurred speech
- Finding it hard to concentrate
- Problems with memory
- Being wobbly on your feet
- Blurred vision
- Feeling sick.

Current best practice

The NICE (2014) Quality Standard indicates that when a person is being treated for anxiety, all care should start with an assessment, which covers the severity of the experience and how it is impacting on the person's life. The first-line response should be the offer of a psychological intervention, and although medicines may also be offered, a benzodiazepine or antipsychotic should not be used without a clear and specific indication for this form of treatment. Each person receiving treatment for anxiety should also have their experience of and response to treatment discussed with them at each session and this should be recorded.

NICE (2019) specifies further that the first-line approach should be a low-intensity psychological intervention, and the second line a higher-intensity psychological intervention and consideration of the use of medication, depending on the person's presentation and preferences. NICE suggests considering an SSRI antidepressant medication first, and states that benzodiazepines must only be used as a short-term intervention. Any use of antipsychotic medication should not take place outside of specialist secondary mental health care.

It is also of note that use of many of the antidepressant medications to support anxiety are, although effective, what we call 'off label' or 'off licence' (i.e. this is not what the medicine was originally set up and licensed to be used for). The antidepressants that are licensed for treatment of anxiety and are used commonly are fluoxetine and venlafaxine, although SSRIs and SNRIs have known efficacy and are also used.

THE MEDICINES LIST

This medicines list will cover the most commonly used medicines in the treatment of anxiety and panic. It is not an exhaustive list and, as mentioned, there are other specialist pathways that may be used by experts in this field.

The medicines list divides medicines into the classifications outlined in this chapter: benzodiazepines, sleeping aids, beta blockers and antidepressants.

Benzodiazepines

The key side effects of benzodiazepines are drowsiness, dizziness, headaches, problems getting an erection, feeling wobbly on your feet, feeling generally unwell and a feeling of weakness in your muscles. If they are given in high doses, benzodiazepines can also affect the respiratory system. This is discussed further in Chapter 6.

Drug name: **Lorazepam**

UK brand names: Ativan

Average doses:

- Oral: 0.5–1 mg per day
- Total maximum within 24 hours: 4mg

What form does it come in? Tablet, solution for emergency injection

Does it interact with any other medications? Yes. The following interactions are known:

- *All antipsychotic medication*: Taking any antipsychotic alongside lorazepam can increase **sedation**
- *Mirtazapine*: Taking mirtazapine alongside lorazepam can increase sedation
- *Tricyclic antidepressants*: Taking any tricyclic antidepressants alongside lorazepam can increase sedative effects
- *Valproate*: Valproate is known to increase the blood level of lorazepam
- *Clozapine:* There is a significant concern that if someone on clozapine takes lorazepam respiratory arrest is more likely, a drop in blood pressure is likely and cardiac arrest is more likely

Drug name: **Clonazepam**

UK brand names: Rivotril

Average doses:

- Oral: 0.5–4mg per day
- Total maximum within 24 hours: 10mg

(Continued)

What form does it come in? Tablet and liquid

Does it interact with any other medications? Yes. The following interactions are known:

- *All antipsychotic medication*: Taking any antipsychotic alongside clonazepam can increase sedation
- *Valproate*: Valproate can increase the blood level of clonazepam
- *Carbamazepine*: Carbamazepine can increase the blood level of clonazepam
- *Lithium*: If clonazepam is taken alongside lithium, there is an increased risk of severe side effects

Drug name: Diazepam

UK brand names: Dialar, Diazemuls, Diazepam Desitin, Diazepam Rectubes, Rimapam, Stesolid, Tensium

Average doses:

- Oral: 2–10mg per day
- Total maximum within 24 hours: 30mg

What form does it come in? Tablet, liquid, solution for injection, rectal tubes. Only tablet and liquid forms are suitable for treatment of anxiety.

Does it interact with any other medications? Yes. The following interactions are known:

- *All antipsychotic medication*: Taking any antipsychotic alongside diazepam can increase sedation
- *Mirtazapine*: Taking mirtazapine alongside diazepam can increase sedation
- *Tricyclic antidepressants*: Taking any tricyclic antidepressants alongside diazepam can increase sedative effects
- *Fluvoxamine*: Fluvoxamine can increase the blood level of diazepam
- *Zotepine*: Zotepine can increase the blood level of diazepam
- *Valproate*: Valproate can increase the blood level of diazepam

- *Clozapine*: There is a significant concern that if someone on clozapine takes diazepam, respiratory arrest is more likely, a drop in blood pressure is likely and cardiac arrest is more likely
- *Olanzapine*: Giving olanzapine and diazepam together creates a risk of slow breathing, slow heartbeat and low blood pressure

Additional information: Diazepam can also be used for alcohol withdrawal

---

***Drug name:* Temazepam** - controlled drug (see Chapter 4)

UK brand names: None

Average doses: Oral: 10–40mg per day

What form does it come in? Tablet and liquid

Does it interact with any other medications? Yes. The following interactions are known:

- *All antipsychotic medication*: Taking any antipsychotic alongside temazepam can increase sedation
- *Mirtazapine*: Taking mirtazapine alongside temazepam can increase sedation
- *Tricyclic antidepressants*: Taking any tricyclic antidepressants alongside temazepam can increase sedative effects
- *Fluvoxamine*: Fluvoxamine can increase the blood level of temazepam
- *Zotepine*: Zotepine can increase the blood level of temazepam
- *Valproate*: Valproate can increase the blood level of temazepam
- *Clozapine*: There is a significant concern that if someone on clozapine takes temazepam respiratory arrest is more likely, a drop in blood pressure is likely and cardiac arrest is more likely
- *Olanzapine*: Giving olanzapine and temazepam together creates a risk of slow breathing, slow heartbeat and low blood pressure
- *Medicines to lower blood pressure*: Temazepam must not be given alongside any medicines that are prescribed to lower blood pressure

(Continued)

Additional information:

- Should only be taken at night
- Should not be taken by people with kidney and liver problems
- Often used as a sleeping aid
- Highly addictive. Treated as a controlled drug since June 2015
- Alcohol must not be consumed
- Cannot drive whilst taking temazepam
- Must not be taken during pregnancy

Sleeping aids ('z' medications)

All sleeping medications should only be taken in the evening, before the person taking the medicine is ready to go to bed. It is really important to work on good sleep hygiene and routines with anyone who is taking medication to help with sleep.

Some of the key common side effects associated with taking the 'z' medications for sleep include a dry mouth, a bitter or metallic taste in the mouth, drowsiness during the daytime, nightmares, headaches, feelings of nausea and feeling an increase in agitation.

Drug name: **Zopiclone**

UK brand names: Zimovane

Average doses: 3.75–7.5mg per day

What form does it come in? Tablet

Does it interact with any other medications? Yes. The following interactions are known:

- *Antipsychotics*: Taking zopiclone with any known antipsychotic may increase the sedating effects
- *Antidepressants*: Taking zopiclone with any known antidepressant may increase the sedating effects

- *Benzodiazepines*: Taking zopiclone with any benzodiazepine may increase the sedating effects
- *Erythromycin antibiotic*: Zopiclone should not be taken with the antibiotic erythromycin, as this can make side effects more likely
- *Medicines for epilepsy*: Medicines for epilepsy such as carbamazepine can make zopiclone less effective

Additional information:

- Should not be taken by anyone with liver, kidney or breathing problems
- Must not be taken with alcohol
- At least seven to eight hours of sleep per night are recommended
- Activities requiring full mental alertness such as driving should not take place within 12 hours of taking the dose

***Drug name*: Zolpidem**

UK brand names: Stilnoct

Average doses: 5–10mg per day

What form does it come in? Tablet

Does it interact with any other medications? Yes. The following interactions are known:

- *Antipsychotics*: Taking zolpidem with any known antipsychotic may increase the sedating effects
- *Antidepressants*: Taking zolpidem with any known antidepressant may increase the sedating effects and can cause an increased risk of suffering hallucinations
- *Benzodiazepines*: Taking zolpidem with any benzodiazepine may increase the sedating effects
- *Erythromycin antibiotic*: Zolpidem should not be taken with the antibiotic erythromycin as this can make side effects more likely
- *St John's wort*: Zolpidem can be less effective if taken with St John's wort
- *Medicines for epilepsy*: Medicines for epilepsy such as carbamazepine can make zolpidem less effective

(Continued)

- *Rifampicin antibiotic*: The antibiotic rifampicin can make zolpidem less effective

Additional information:

- Should not be taken by anyone with liver, kidney or breathing problems
- Must not be taken with alcohol
- At least seven to eight hours of sleep per night are recommended
- Activities requiring full mental alertness such as driving should not take place within 12 hours of taking the dose

Beta blockers

A full cardiac history and assessment is required before you can consider commencing a person with anxiety on a beta blocker medication. They should not be used in people with a low blood pressure or low heart rate.

Some of the common side effects noted with beta blockers include a low heart rate, low blood pressure, cold fingers and toes, constipation, gastro-intestinal disturbances, feeling tired and sweating more than usual.

Drug name: **Propranolol**

UK brand names: Bedranol

Average doses: 10-80mg, up to three times a day. Can be taken one hour before an anticipated stressful event

What form does it come in? Tablet

Does it interact with any other medications? Yes. The following interactions are known:

- *Calcium channel blockers*: Propranolol should not be prescribed to anyone taking a calcium channel blocker (e.g. verapamil)
- *Asthma*: It should not be given to anyone with asthma as it can prevent the effect of bronchodilators
- *Warfarin*: Caution must be used in people taking warfarin

- *Fluvoxamine*: Propranolol should not be taken with fluvoxamine as this can cause a severely low heart rate
- *Chlorpromazine*: Propranolol should not be taken with chlorpromazine as this can cause a severely low heart rate and blood pressure

Additional information:

- Should not be prescribed for anyone with chronic obstructive pulmonary disease (COPD)
- Tablets contain lactose
- Caution to be taken for people with liver and kidney disease

---

***Drug name*: Atenolol**

UK brand names: Tenormin

Average doses: 50-100mg once daily

What form does it come in? Tablet and liquid

Does it interact with any other medications? Yes. The following interactions are known:

- *Calcium channel blockers*: Atenolol should not be prescribed to anyone taking a calcium channel blocker (e.g. verapamil)
- *Diabetes*: Caution should be used in people with diabetes. If taken with atenolol, the blood sugar lowering effects of insulin and oral antidiabetic drugs can be increased

Additional information: Can be highly toxic in overdose

Antidepressants

For an exhaustive list of SSRI medications and side effects see Chapter 1.

(Continued)

Other medications

Drug name: Pregabalin

UK brand names: Lyrica, Alzain, Lecaent and Rewisca

Average doses: Maximum of 600mg daily (once titrated) in two to three divided doses

What form does it come in? Tablet

Does it interact with any other medications? Yes. People taking this medication should be informed of the potentially fatal risks of interactions between pregabalin and alcohol, and with other medicines that cause central nervous system depression, particularly opioids

Additional information: Pregabalin has been a class C controlled substance since April 2019 and may not be suitable for those with substance misuse histories. Pregabalin is also linked to a risk of respiratory depression and so caution is advised in those over 65, those with a compromised respiratory function, respiratory or neurological disease or a renal impairment

Drug name: Buspirone

UK brand names: Buspar

Average dose: Usually 15-30mg daily, with a maximum of 45mg daily in divided doses

What form does it come in? Tablet (5mg and 10mg)

Does it interact with any other medications? Yes. If a person is also taking a benzodiazepine it is helpful if they can be withdrawn from this before starting buspirone

Additional information: May not be suitable for people with epilepsy

MEDICINES FOR ANXIETY IN PREGNANT WOMEN AND BREASTFEEDING MOTHERS

It is recommended that tranquillising medications, particularly benzodiazepines, are not given to women who are expectant or new mothers. They are linked with the development of cleft lip and cleft palate in the fetus if they are taken during pregnancy.

If a baby is born to a mother who has been taking tranquillising medication, the baby will need special medical support as it may be at risk of developing withdrawal symptoms. This can be very distressing in the new baby and includes symptoms such as fever, inability to settle, increased sweating, problems sleeping, problems with breathing and feeding, and decreased alertness and responsiveness.

It has been noted that benzodiazepines can accumulate in higher doses in breast milk than they do in the blood stream, and therefore any new mother who is taking such medication would be advised not to breastfeed as these high doses could then be passed onto the baby, who would struggle to tolerate this. However, if you are in a situation where this is being discussed, you need to ensure that you approach it sensitively as the decision not to breastfeed could be very emotive for the new mother, and she may need considerable support when making this decision.

For more about the impact of antidepressants on new and expectant mothers see Chapter 1.

The side effects of pregabalin in pregnancy are not clear: there may be a slightly increased risk of birth defects, especially when taken within the first 12 weeks of pregnancy, but research into this area is still developing.

CONSIDERATIONS FOR DIFFERENT AGE GROUPS

Anxiety can impact all people, across the age span. The NICE (2014) Quality Standard for anxiety recognises that many anxiety disorders can start to appear early in life, and that anxiety disorders in children and young people, if not identified and treated early, may continue into and through adult life, and can also increase risks of depression and substance abuse.

Older adults

In older adults, any physical conditions that may be causing the anxiety must be carefully considered and ruled out (Subramanyam et al., 2018). Psychological interventions can be used, being mindful of the person's level of cognitive functioning. There needs to be very careful consideration of the use of any sedating medications, as these can increase the risk of falls, and using benzodiazepines can also increase agitation in some older adults and so may not be suitable; the person's response to these must closely be monitored.

Children and young people

The NICE guidelines (2013) for treating anxiety in children and young people state that medication should not routinely be offered as a treatment, and the focus should be on access to psychological therapies, usually individual or group CBT with children of a similar age. Children aged over 15 may access an adult-based therapy, depending on suitability and the child's development. Any use of medicines must be through a specialist service and closely monitored.

LEARNING FROM A CASE STUDY: TEST YOUR KNOWLEDGE

Susie is 19 years old and has been having a difficult time in her personal life. She has recently left home for the first time and is struggling with being away from home and managing her finances. She has recently broken up with her boyfriend and has also fallen out with her best friend as she does not have enough money to socialise. Susie is working extra hours to try to keep up with her finances. This is making her feel stressed and she is not sleeping properly. She has started having panic attacks and is convinced that she is going to have a heart attack and die on the bus to work. She feels anxious all the time, with worries going round and round in her head all day and night. Susie therefore decides to see her GP to ask for help. The GP prescribes her a daily dose of diazepam 5mg, and tells her to come back in for a review in three months' time.

1 What sort of medication is diazepam?
2 What is your concern about the GP asking Susie to come back in three months' time?
3 What else should the GP have done during his initial appointment with Susie?

After taking the diazepam 5mg daily for seven weeks, Susie finds out that she is pregnant, and so she decides to stop taking the medication with immediate effect as she is worried that it may harm her baby.

4 What is the concern with Susie suddenly stopping her medication? How should this be managed?
5 If Susie were to continue to take the diazepam during her pregnancy, what may be the concerns?

IF I REMEMBER 5 THINGS FROM THIS CHAPTER ...

1. Benzodiazepines are highly addictive and should only be used on a short-term basis, ideally for no more than four weeks.
2. Medication is not the only answer for treating anxiety: psychological interventions are often the most effective treatment in this area.
3. There are both long-acting and short-acting forms of benzodiazepines.
4. No medication prescribed for anxiety should be stopped suddenly. Instead, people coming off medication should be supported to do this by gradually reducing their dose.
5. Beta blockers are often prescribed to help manage the physical side effects of feeling very anxious, but they do not treat the root cause of the anxiety.

ANSWERS TO THE CASE STUDY QUESTIONS

1. Diazepam is a benzodiazepine medication.
2. Benzodiazepine medication should not be prescribed for longer than four weeks. Therefore, the GP should review Susie before she has been taking the medication for four weeks, ensuring that there is a plan to help her to come off the medication as soon as she is able to. He should also have ensured that she was aware of the possible side effects of the diazepam, the risk of addiction and the risk of withdrawal.
3. The GP should have discussed how medication is a last resort. He should have explored with Susie the reasons for her anxiety and made an immediate referral for Susie to have a psychological intervention such as CBT.
4. If Susie suddenly stops taking her medication, she may be at risk of withdrawal symptoms. She may therefore need to be taken off her diazepam gradually by slowly reducing the dose.
5. Benzodiazepines are linked with the formation of cleft lip and cleft palate defects in unborn babies, and babies of mothers on benzodiazepines are also at risk of withdrawal symptoms when they are born.

REFERENCES AND RECOMMENDED READING

Groves, P. (2016) 'Mindfulness in psychiatry: Where are we at now?', *British Journal of Psychiatry Bulletin*, 40 (6): 289–92. Available at: www.ncbi.nlm. nih.gov/pmc/articles/PMC5353527 (last accessed 29 September 2021).

Mind (2021) 'Psychiatric medication: An alphabetical list'. Available at: www.mind.org.uk/information-support/drugs-and-treatments/medication/drug-names-a-z/ (accessed 11 June 2017).

NHS (2016) 'Mindfulness'. Available at: www.nhs.uk/Conditions/stress-anxiety-depression/Pages/mindfulness.aspx (accessed 19 December 2017).

NICE (2013) 'Social anxiety disorder: Recognition, assessment and treatment: Treatment for children and young people'. Available at www.nice.org.uk/guidance/cg159/ifp/chapter/treatment-for-children-and-young-people (accessed 30 June 2021).

NICE (2014) 'Anxiety disorders: Quality Standard 53'. Available at www.nice.org.uk/guidance/qs53 (accessed 30 June 2021).

NICE (2019) 'Generalised anxiety disorder and panic disorder in adults: Management'. Available at www.nice.org.uk/guidance/cg113 (accessed 30 June 2021).

Richards, T.A. (2016) 'Basic facts about panic attacks'. Available at: https://anxietynetwork.com/content/basic-facts-panic-attacks (accessed 11 June 2017).

Royal College of Psychiatrists (2013) 'Benzodiazepines'. Available at: www.rcpsych.ac.uk/healthadvice/treatmentswellbeing/benzodiazepines.aspx (accessed 11 June 2017).

Royal College of Psychiatrists (2014) 'Anxiety, panic and phobias'. Available at: www.rcpsych.ac.uk/mental-health/problems-disorders/anxiety-panic-and-phobias (accessed 11 June 2017).

Strauss, C., Cavanaugh, K., Oliver, A., et al. (2014) 'Mindfulness-based interventions for people diagnosed with a current episode of an anxiety or depressive disorder: A meta-analysis of randomised controlled trials'. London: NHS, National Institute for Health Research. Available at: www.crd.york.ac.uk/crdweb/ShowRecord.asp?LinkFrom=OAI&ID=12014028944 (accessed 11 June 2017).

Subramanyam, A., Kedare, J., Singh, O.P., et al. (2018) 'Clinical practice guidelines for geriatric anxiety disorders'. *Indian Journal of Psychiatry*, 60 (3): 371–82.

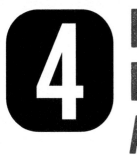

4 MEDICINES FOR ALCOHOL AND DRUG DEPENDENCE

EMILY FLOYD

AFTER READING THIS CHAPTER, YOU WILL BE ABLE TO:

- Define what the term **dependence** means
- Understand some of the factors that contribute to the development of an addiction or dependence
- Demonstrate an awareness of different types of substances that people may become dependent on
- Be aware of possible interventions for different types of dependence
- Describe the concept of 'recovery'
- Think about how substance abuse and consequent treatment may impact on pregnant and breastfeeding mothers

---

SUBSTANCE ABUSE AND MENTAL HEALTH

Within any given year, mental health illness affects one in four people in the UK (McManus et al., 2009). When we consider this statistic along with the estimated figure of two million people in the UK suffering from addiction (NHS, 2021) we must acknowledge that for many they are coexisting health problems. Individuals who are living with depression might use a substance such as cocaine to relieve and manage their symptoms, or those suffering with anxiety might use cannabis to 'relax' them. We must consider the impact that both forms of illness can have on service users and must acknowledge that many people living with a mental health illness could also be living with substance addiction. Data is showing increases in the number of people now receiving support with drug and alcohol issues, and the trends are also changing, with a particular increase in the use of crack cocaine (Public Health England, 2019). This data also highlights the severity of the impact of living with these challenges; 1.1 per cent of people die whilst in contact with a treatment service, and in England, the number of deaths from drug misuse registered in 2018 increased by 16 per cent to 2,670. This is the highest level ever, with deaths of middle-aged heroin users being one of the main causes of the increase in drug poisonings. There was also a large increase in deaths involving powder cocaine or crack.

With the world now recovering from COVID-19, we are seeing even more of an increase in those living with substance misuse issues, as people have higher rates of trauma, anxiety and depression, have been lonely and socially isolated and have not had access to other coping mechanisms (Abramson, 2021).

The link between substance abuse and health inequalities also needs to be considered, with poverty, income and social deprivation increasing individual risks of developing challenges with substance misuse. The most recent statistics on drug misuse in England (NHS Digital, 2020) showed that admissions to hospital for drug-related mental and behavioural disorders and poisoning related to drug misuse are five times higher in areas of the highest levels of social deprivation (compared to the least deprived areas), and admissions to hospital where the primary or secondary diagnosis was a drug-related mental or behavioural disorder were over eight times more likely in these areas of high social deprivation. Public Health England (2019) show that around one-fifth of those receiving support with drug and alcohol use are having challenges with their housing and over half also have another mental health treatment need.

WHAT IS DEPENDENCE?

When we consider dependence in relation to substance abuse, it is essential to understand what we mean by this term. 'Dependence' describes the inability to have control over doing something and makes the concept of 'choice' in decision-making very difficult, therefore creating an addiction.

There is a false view that people who suffer from addiction cannot function in society – in other words they can't hold down a job, form meaningful relationships or care for themselves. However, there are many forms of addiction. Some people are addicted to nicotine on a level that is not debilitating in terms of functioning in society. There is also the term 'functioning alcoholics' referring to those who considerably exceed the daily recommended alcohol intake but wouldn't necessarily class themselves as 'alcoholics' and maintain a 'functioning' lifestyle within society. However, many individuals addicted to substances such as illicit drugs and alcohol are impacted so heavily that they can no longer live a life that they find meaningful or fulfilling. The implications of being addicted to a substance or substances affect so many facets of the life of individuals: family life, forming and maintaining relationships, physical health, mental health and work life.

WHY DO PEOPLE BECOME ADDICTED TO SUBSTANCES?

Dopamine is a neurotransmitter that is involved in our pleasure and reward system. We know that when we are doing something we enjoy, the levels of dopamine in the brain's pleasure centre increase. When this act is repeated regularly, the continual surge of dopamine levels in the pleasure centre makes it pleasing: the act could be practising hobbies, having sex, eating – indeed, anything that an individual takes pleasure from. The use of drugs and alcohol, however, creates an associated surge in dopamine levels around two to ten times greater (NIDA, 2016), and this results in a feeling of great enjoyment (Di Chiara et al., 1998).

Once an individual has released this larger amount of dopamine, experiencing the pleasure and reward, it becomes more difficult to re-create. Therefore, many people practise the act more frequently and in greater volumes, meaning that an individual's 'tolerance' builds. By repeating the same act, the resulting higher levels of dopamine soon become 'normal' to the brain and the ability for the individual to experience any pleasure from 'normal rewards' becomes compromised. Hence, this leads to the development of an addiction.

When we look at the causes of addiction, social influences are also important. Factors such as stressful jobs and lifestyles can lead individuals to seek a form of escapism through substances. A desire for social acceptance and learned behaviours might also contribute to an individual's decision to take substances, and so might the occurrence of traumatic life events. There are also theories and studies to support a genetic argument for addiction, suggesting that it can be an inherent disease and traced through family history.

RECOVERY IN MENTAL HEALTH AND ADDICTION SERVICES

'Recovery' is a frequently used term. It was originally used in the area of addiction to describe an individual who is in recovery from substance abuse. The concept encourages empowerment for the service user to take a lead in their care planning and delivery, enabling us as healthcare professionals to support, educate and facilitate. When an individual is embarking on a journey of **abstinence**, we should avoid sole focus on the pharmacological aspect of treatment and engage and encourage the emotional and psychological aspects of the person's recovery journey.

ALCOHOL DEPENDENCE

With alcohol considered to be one of the most addictive and widely available drugs in society (Preedy, 2016), it is easy to understand how those living with mental illness become addicted to it and how those addicted to alcohol develop symptoms of mental illness. Comorbidity between alcohol dependence and mental illness is extremely common.

Advice and self-diagnostic tests are readily available for individuals to monitor their alcohol consumption and are developed in line with the government's *Low Risk Drinking Guidelines* (DH, 2016), which recommends no more than 14 units of alcohol per week. Alcohol dependence and abuse are regarded as a very high priority public health concern, with as many as 10.8 million adults in England drinking at levels that can pose some risk to their health and 1.6 million of these having a dependence on alcohol (Public Health England, 2016).

Settings for alcohol detox

In the current climate of available mental health services and resources, alcohol detox programmes are most commonly found within the private sector. However, the comorbidity of alcohol abuse and mental illness will see many individuals as an inpatient in acute mental health services. During these admissions, service users will be assessed for their level of dependence on alcohol and the risk of the withdrawal symptoms they might experience. A detox regime will be prescribed in accordance with this assessment.

Signs and symptoms of alcohol withdrawal

When we consider the nurse's role in the assessment of a person's response to the treatment of alcohol detoxification, healthcare professionals must be extremely vigilant in monitoring potentially life-threatening symptoms.

Common physical symptoms are:

- Nausea and vomiting
- Shakes and tremors

- Clammy skin and sweating
- Dizziness
- Headaches
- Sickness and diarrhoea
- Dehydration
- Loss of appetite
- Pupil dilation
- **Insomnia**.

Mood and emotional responses are:

- Irritability
- Anxiety
- Rapid changes in mood
- Low mood
- Thoughts of harming self
- Thoughts of suicide.

If not monitored closely and not treated, the impact of these withdrawal symptoms can be life-threatening. Vital signs should be monitored closely and intervals adjusted accordingly to meet the presentation of the service user. The multidisciplinary team should be informed of any changes or concerns based on the person's physical or mental health so that appropriate formulation and care planning can be devised.

Critical conditions are:

- ***Delirium*** *tremens*: This is a severe response to alcohol withdrawal that severely affects changes in the mental and/or nervous system. Individuals might experience hallucinations, severe confusion, fever and withdrawal seizures.
- *Withdrawal seizures*: These are most likely to be 'tonic-clonic seizures' and mostly occur within the first 12–48 hours after the last ingestion of alcohol. They are most common in individuals who have experienced serious effects of withdrawal in the past and affect the whole of the brain. These typically last for about two to three minutes. They are characterised by stiffness and rigidity of muscles, and loss of consciousness – with a potential to bite their tongue.
- *Wernicke's encephalopathy*: This is due to a lack of vitamin B1 and causes brain damage, affecting the thalamus and hypothalamus. Individuals might experience tremors due to a lack of muscle coordination and problems with vision – they can experience double vision and involuntary eye movements.

- *Korsakoff's syndrome*: This condition is a form of Alzheimer's disease and classed as a dementia. It also occurs due to brain damage (lack of vitamin B1) and often as a result of Wernicke's encephalopathy. Individuals might experience severe memory loss, poor short-term memory and hallucinations.

It is essential to note that many of the signs and symptoms of alcohol withdrawal can easily be mistaken as behaviours and characteristics of mental illness and vice versa. As previously discussed, many service users will have a dual diagnosis or coexisting illness, making it crucial for them to have a thorough risk assessment, clinical decision-making and effective treatment plans.

The use of benzodiazepines in managing the symptoms of alcohol withdrawal

Benzodiazepines are the most commonly prescribed drugs when treating alcohol abuse and dependence and are recommended for first-line treatment (WHO, 2012). The use of these medications is considered to be the most effective in minimising the experience of withdrawal and service users are prescribed a regime lasting three to seven days on average, depending on the level of their alcohol abuse. However, it is important that these are prescribed for short-term use in alcohol withdrawal and closely monitored because evidence suggests that medications in this drug group can be highly addictive in long-term use.

The most common side effects of benzodiazepine use include drowsiness, confusion, amnesia, dependence, dizziness, muscle weakness/involuntary movements and **respiratory depression**.

THE MEDICINES LIST

This medicines list presents the key medicines used to treat alcohol dependence, medicines used for smoking cessation and medicines used to support treatment of drug dependencies.

Drug name: Chlordiazepoxide hydrochloride

UK brand names: None known

Average doses: 10–50mg four times daily

What form does it come in? Capsule and tablet

Does it interact with any other medicines? Yes. The following interactions are known:

- *Aripiprazole, citalopram, escitalopram and pregabalin*: Chlordiazepoxide hydrochloride can increase drowsiness and sedative effects and affect concentration when taken with aripiprazole, citalopram, escitalopram and pregabalin

Caution:

- Tasks that require concentration such as driving should be avoided
- Short-term use due to high risk of dependence

Drug name: Diazepam

UK brand names: Dialaer, Diazemuls, Diazepam Desitin, Diazepam Rectubes, Rimapam, Stesolid, Tensium

Average doses: 5mg four times daily

What form does it come in? Tablet, injection, rectal tube, suppository, oral solution

Does it interact with any other medicines? Yes. The following interactions are known:

- *Duloxetine, escitalopram and quetiapine*: Diazepam can increase drowsiness and sedative effects and affect concentration when taken with duloxetine, escitalopram and quetiapine

Caution:

- Tasks that require concentration such as driving should be avoided
- Short-term use due to high risk of dependence

Drug name: Oxazepam - used in cases when the liver is severely damaged

UK brand names: None known

Average doses: 15-30mg three to four times daily

(Continued)

What form does it come in? Tablet

Does it interact with any other medicines? Yes. The following interactions are known:

- *Aripiprazole, duloxetine, escitalopram, pregabalin, quetiapine, sertraline and venlafaxine*: Oxazepam can increase drowsiness and sedative effects and affect concentration when taken with aripiprazole, duloxetine, escitalopram, pregabalin, quetiapine, sertraline and venlafaxine

Caution:

- Tasks that require concentration such as driving should be avoided
- Short-term use due to high risk of dependence

Other medicines used

Drug name: Acamprosate – prescribed for maintenance after the patient has achieved abstinence; most effective in conjunction with counselling

UK brand names: Campral

Average doses: 666mg three times daily

What form does it come in? Tablet

Common side effects: Nausea and vomiting, diarrhoea, changes in libido, feeling itchy, developing a rash

Does it interact with any other medicines? Yes. The following interactions are known:

- *Naltrexone* can increase levels of acamprosate

Caution:

- Treatment will be ineffective if alcohol consumption continues

Drug name: Disulfiram – creates unpleasant reaction if alcohol is ingested, including nausea and vomiting, diarrhoea, headaches, hot flushes, **tachycardia**

UK brand names: Antabuse

Average doses: A one-off initial dose of 800mg, reducing over five days to approximately 100–200mg daily

What form does it come in? Tablet

Common side effects: Nausea and vomiting, fatigue, drowsiness, reduction in libido, halitosis

Does it interact with any other medicines? Yes. The following interactions are known:

- *Can increase the sedative effects of*: Clonazepam, diazepam, lorazepam
- *Sertraline oral solution*: Contains alcohol, therefore it is not recommended for prescription

Caution:

- Do not administer if alcohol has been ingested within 12 hours. Any products containing even a small amount of alcohol are to be avoided
- Has been known to provoke or induce symptoms of mania, depression, paranoia and schizophrenia

Drug name: Carbamazepine – used off-licence as an alternative to benzodiazepines if they are not tolerated, in acute alcohol withdrawal

UK brand names: Tegretol, Carbagen SR, Tegretol Retard

Average doses: 800mg daily in split doses, gradual reduction over five days to 200mg daily

What form does it come in? Tablet and liquid

Common side effects: Nausea and vomiting, fatigue, drowsiness, headaches, blood disorders, involuntary muscle movement, **oedema**, skin disorders, dry mouth, low sodium levels

(Continued)

Does it interact with any other medicines? Yes. The following interactions are known:

- *Buprenorphine*: Due to the effects on the central nervous system, carbamazepine can cause side effects such as respiratory disease, and induce a coma and death if used with buprenorphine
- *Clozapine*: Carbamazepine can affect blood cell count and bone marrow function if used with clozapine
- *Clonazepam, lamotrigine, quetiapine, valproate*: Carbamazepine can alter blood levels and the effectiveness of both drugs if used with clonazepam, lamotrigine, quetiapine, valproate

Caution:

- Can exacerbate or trigger psychosis, depressed mood and thoughts of self-harm and/or suicide
- Regular blood tests for liver and renal function are required

Drug name: Clomethiazole – should only be used in an inpatient setting and should not be prescribed if the service user is likely to imbibe alcohol. Maximum use of nine days

UK brand names: Heminevrin

Average doses: Initial 2-4 capsules; on day one take 9-12 capsules; on day two take 6-8 capsules; on day three take 4-6 capsules. Gradual reduction over days four to six; and doses to be split around 3-4 separate doses per day

What form does it come in? Capsule

Common side effects: Headaches, nasal and eye irritation

Does it interact with other medicines: Yes. The following interactions are known:

- *Can increase the sedative effects of*: Carbamazepine, citalopram, clozapine, duloxetine, escitalopram, fluoxetine, fluphenazine, haloperidol, methadone, promethazine, risperidone, zuclopenthixol

Caution:

- Avoid prolonged use due to dependence risk
- Monitor for excessive sedation

Drug name: Thiamine or vitamin B1 – used to treat vitamin deficiency and as a preventative measure against Wernicke's encephalopathy. Most effective treatment is three to five days intramuscular (IM) administration, followed by oral

UK brand names: Pabrinex (IM)

Average doses: Oral 100-300mg daily, IM solution (500mg ascorbic acid, 250mg thiamine, nicotinamide 160mg, pyridoxine hydrochloride 50mg, riboflavin 4mg) daily

What form does it come in? Tablet and IM solution

Common side effects of IM: hypotension, feeling of pins and needles, discomfort at site of injection

Does it interact with other medicines? There are no known interactions

Caution:

- IM preparation of full dose requires 2 ampules for a full 7ml dose combination
- IM preparation must be stored in an appropriate refrigerator for medicines at 2-8°C
- IM in some cases has caused anaphylaxis after prolonged doses of administration

NICOTINE

People living with a long-term mental health problem are twice as likely to be smokers (Mental Health Taskforce Strategy, 2016).

With many trusts implementing a 'smoke free' policy, smoking-cessation education and services are paramount when providing our service users with support, holistic care and considering informed decision-making. In our role as nurses, skills in health promotion are essential.

Most individuals access smoking-cessation support through primary care services. However, in relation to mental health services, NICE (2013: 68) recommends providing 'intensive support for people using acute and mental health services' with facilities to support and educate service users around smoking choices and alternatives.

Some service users might commence nicotine replacement therapy whilst an inpatient in mental health services: as a nurse administering prescribed medications, do familiarise yourself with the service user's cessation treatment plan and be mindful of whether the service user is still smoking cigarettes before administering anything containing nicotine.

In relation to smoking it is also important to be aware that changes in the amount a person smokes can impact on some medications and how they are absorbed by the body. Clozapine (an antipsychotic) is one medication in particular where the person's clozapine level is impacted by their smoking. Please see Chapter 5 for a specialist section on this.

SIGNS AND SYMPTOMS OF NICOTINE WITHDRAWAL

Common physical experiences:

- An increase in appetite
- Weight gain
- Headaches
- Dizziness
- Coughing
- Flu-like symptoms.

Mood and emotional responses:

- Poor sleep
- Irritability
- Depression
- Anxiety
- Poor concentration
- Restlessness.

As smoking can affect the metabolic rate of some medications, it is essential to note that the dosage of the following antipsychotic medications must be reviewed and altered accordingly in circumstances where a service user has reduced their smoking intake or stopped smoking altogether:

- Clozapine
- Chlorpromazine
- Haloperidol
- Olanzapine.

This is crucial, as it ensures that the correct **therapeutic dose** is being administered and that the service user is not at risk of overdose and potentially life-threatening conditions.

NICOTINE REPLACEMENT THERAPY (NRT)

Evidence suggests that by using nicotine replacement therapy (NRT) to help quit smoking, an individual's chance of success is about 50–70 per cent (Stead et al., 2012). By administering doses of nicotine, there is a reduction in the individual's experience of cravings. The most common stock preparation(s) for NRT are administered by the following routes and are in the following forms:

- Oral: Inhalators
- Oral: Lozenges
- Oral: Chewing gum
- Oral: Sublingual tablets
- Topical: Nasal spray
- Topical: Transdermal skin patch.

UK brand names: Nicorette, Nicotinell, NiQuitin

Table 4.1 provides guidance for each stock preparation. However, do check the prescription and the recommendations for each brand thoroughly before administration as these factors can vary considerably.

Table 4.1 Stock preparation guidance

Preparation	Dose	Common side effects	Drug interactions	Caution(s)
		Transferable among all		
Inhalator	Up to 12 cartridges per day, for use PRN	- Heartburn - Nausea - Diarrhoea - Indigestion	- Bupropion; can cause an increase in heart rate potentially leading to hypertension	- Monitor cigarette consumption to avoid overdose - Do not apply patches to broken skin

(Continued)

Table 4.1   (Continued)

Preparation	Dose	Common side effects	Drug interactions	Caution(s)
Lozenges	One lozenge 1-2 hourly No more than 15 in 24 hours Use lower strength lozenges for individuals smoking <20 cigarettes per day	- Congested nose - Coughing - Sore throat - Headache - Sore mouth - Stomach ache/pain	- Varenicline; nausea and vomiting, headaches and fatigue	- Acidic drinks can impact absorption of nicotine, avoid 15 minutes before administration
Chewing gum	< 20 cigarettes per day use one piece of 2mg gum PRN. No more than 15 pieces daily. However, if more pieces required or smoke >20 cigarettes per day, 4mg gum	- Fatigue - Flu-like symptoms - Sweating - Rash - Taste alteration - Dry mouth - Excessive wind - Constipation - Hypertension	- Naltrexone: can cause an increase in heart rate potentially leading to hypotension	- Stop using the gum and speak to a doctor if you have any mouth, teeth or jaw problems
Sublingual tablets	<20 cigarettes per day, initiate 1 tablet hourly, can increase to 2 if required. >20 cigarettes per day, 2 tablets hourly Maximum 40 tablets per day	- Restlessness - Anxiety - Irritability - Disturbed sleep - Labile mood - Low mood	None	None
Nasal spray	Use 1 spray in each nostril PRN Up to 2 every hour (based on 16 waking hours) maximum 64 sprays	None	None	None
Skin patch	Do not exceed 1 patch in 24 hours	None	None	None

THE MEDICINES LIST

***Drug name:* Bupropion** – commence treatment one to two weeks prior to quit date

UK brand names: Zyban

Average doses: For the first six days, 150mg daily, then 150mg twice daily for about eight weeks. Maximum dose 300mg daily with eight hours between doses

What form does it come in? Tablet

Common side effects: Disturbed vision, dry mouth, headaches, stomach ache, poor sleep, tremors, feeling itchy, developing a rash, flu-like symptoms, dizziness, poor concentration, low mood, anxiety

Does it interact with any other medicines? Yes. The following interactions are known:

- *Other medications*: Can increase the risk of seizures and increase the blood levels of some medications including amitriptyline, aripiprazole, buprenorphine, chlordiazepoxide, citalopram, clomipramine, clozapine, donepezil, duloxetine, fluoxetine, ibuprofen, lithium, methadone, mirtazapine, morphine, naltrexone, olanzapine, promethazine, risperidone
- Monitor blood pressure prior to and throughout treatment
- Can cause a seizure if used when experiencing alcohol and/or benzodiazepine withdrawal

***Drug name:* Varenicline** – commence treatment one to two weeks prior to quit date

UK brand names: Champix

Average doses: Commence 500mcg once daily for first three days, increase to 500mcg twice daily for next four days, then 1mg twice daily for 11 weeks

What form does it come in? Tablet

Common side effects: Stomach ache, dry mouth, taste alterations, poor sleep, nausea, headaches

(Continued)

Does it interact with any other medicines? Yes. The following interactions are known:

- *NRT*: Can increase side effects if using nicotine replacement therapy

Caution:

- Patients with a history of mental illness must be closely monitored due to the risk of an increase in low mood, suicidal ideation and poor sleep

Along with medical interventions, there are also talking therapies available, such as regular appointments with a smoking-cessation professional to discuss progress and set targets such as quit teas, self-rewards and the effectiveness of the prescribed NRT (if any). Some group activities are also available to provide support networks and smoking education.

OPIATES AND OPIOIDS

Heroin is a drug that is derived from morphine and is considered to be one of the most addictive substances available. It has an extremely powerful sedative and pain relief effect and is commonly used by those who are suffering from mental health problems and other forms of substance misuse.

Heroin users generally smoke, snort or inject the drug intravenously (IV). By using the IV method to take heroin, the individual can immediately expose themselves to physical health risks such as damage to veins, needle-stick injuries and exposure to infection. The risk of exposure to infection not only comes from the injection site, or the contents of the drug itself, but also from sharing needles and sharps used to take the drug. HIV and hepatitis C are a widespread concern for individuals sharing needles as the virus is passed through infected bloods and/or bodily fluids.

Heroin detox

In the UK, there are two main forms of heroin addiction treatments, with methadone and buprenorphine used as the substitute medication therapy.

Substitution therapies are regularly prescribed doses of alternative opiate medication administered by a healthcare professional. As this is generally a long-term approach to dependence and/or reduction, service users access this prescription through their local primary healthcare services. For example, daily clinics are run in pharmacy settings to administer these doses, ensuring that the service user maintains a safe level of the drug in their system in order to stick to their regime.

Withdrawal regime

This consists of a reduction programme aiming for the service user to achieve abstinence from the drug. The regime will be prescribed for about four weeks in an inpatient setting and for about 12 weeks in the community. The service user will initially be introduced to the chosen opiate substitute and a period of stabilisation will be achieved prior to reduction.

As with all drug administration, there are risks. In the case of opiate substitute medication, there is a possibility of relapse and potential for the service user to self-administer heroin or other illicit/non-prescribed medications. The tolerance of heroin by individuals who are on substitution therapy also decreases dramatically, so fatalities are common in relapse periods – previous amounts of heroin that were used will no longer be tolerable. It is essential that monitoring for signs of this behaviour is carried out and acted upon accordingly in order to avoid any overdose or risk of toxicity.

Self-administration of opiate substitution medication(s) is prescribed in small doses; however, the following factors are considered:

- Service user's compliance with treatment plan
- Risk of overdose
- Risk of using heroin
- History of non-compliance with services
- Physical health concerns
- Vulnerability.

Opiate substitution medication is a 'controlled drug' (CD). This means that local guidance must be followed in relation to controlled drug policy and practice.

Signs and symptoms of opiate withdrawal

Signs of withdrawal from heroin occur about 8–12 hours after its last use and, within two days, these symptoms become severe. After about five days, withdrawal symptoms decrease dramatically. However, due to the severe discomfort and rapid onset of these symptoms, it is extremely difficult for individuals to embark on reduction therapy and/or detox.

Common physical experiences:

- Nausea and vomiting
- Shakes and tremors
- Chills and cold sweats
- Sneezing
- Itchy skin
- Diarrhoea
- Cramping
- Excessive yawning
- Pain in bones and muscle
- Insomnia.

Mood and emotional response:

- Extreme agitation
- Anxiety
- Low mood.

Opiate substitutes

Methadone and buprenorphine are the medications used for opiate substitution therapy. The most common side effects caused by these medications are nausea, vomiting, diarrhoea, constipation, stomach ache, headache, dry mouth, muscle stiffness, hypotension, **bradycardia**, tachycardia, **heart palpitations**, oedema, dizziness, confusion, retention of urine, sweating, development of rash, hot flushes, poor sleep, sexual dysfunction, drowsiness, dependence, respiratory depression, confusion, erratic mood – **euphoria** and **dysphoria**.

Note that there are extreme similarities between the signs and symptoms of withdrawal from the drug itself and the side effects of treatment.

THE MEDICINES LIST

Drug name: **Buprenorphine**

UK brand names: Subutex

Average doses: Day one initial dose 0.8-4mg, titrate 2-4mg accordingly until average dose of 12-24mg daily

What form does it come in? Sublingual tablet

Does it interact with any other medicines? Yes. The following interactions are known:

- *Other medications*: This medication should not be used with other medicines that can cause respiratory depression, due to a combined increased risk of coma or death. Such medicines are aripiprazole, bupropion, chlordiazepoxide, chlorpheniramine, citalopram, clonazepam, clozapine, diazepam, fluphenazine, haloperidol, lorazepam, methadone, naltrexone, olanzapine, paliperidone, promethazine, risperidone

Caution:

- Long-term use can cause serious implications and disruption of the sexual function in both males and females, causing such side effects as **impotence** and infertility
- Repeated use is associated with dependence both psychologically and physically

---

Drug name: Methadone

UK brand names: Metharose

Average doses: 60–120mg daily after effective titration period, starting at 10–40mg daily

What form does it come in? Oral solution

Does it interact with any other medicines? Yes. The following interactions are known:

- *Other medications*: Using this medication with some others can cause depression related to the central nervous system such as respiratory depression, induction of a coma or death. These other medications include aripiprazole, bupropion, chlordiazepoxide, chlorpheniramine, citalopran, clonazepam, clozapine, diazepam, fluphenazine, haloperidol, lorazepam, methadone, naltrexone, olanzapine, paliperidone, promethazine, risperidone

(Continued)

Caution:

- Long-term use can cause serious implications and disruption of the sexual function in both males and females, causing such side effects as impotence and infertility
- Repeated use is associated with dependence both psychologically and physically
- Regular ECGs are recommended

As previously discussed, the withdrawal symptoms experienced are extremely severe. We must therefore ensure as healthcare professionals that we not only monitor and support service users psychologically but that we also offer medical interventions where appropriate and possible

The following list can support service users:

- *Paracetamol and ibuprofen*: To ease bodily pain and headaches
- *Loperamide*: To manage symptoms of diarrhoea
- *Mebeverine*: To ease stomach ache and cramps
- *Short-term benzodiazepines or zopiclone*: For support with poor sleep

Drug name: Lofexidine – to minimise withdrawal symptoms, often pre-scribed with opiate-substitute therapy or can be used solely for a mild dependence

UK brand names: BritLofex

Average doses: 2.4mg daily maximum dose, after initial titration from 800mcg daily in divided doses. Do not exceed 800mcg in one dose

What form does it come in? Tablet

Common side effects: Bradycardia, hypotension, dizziness, drowsiness, and dry mucous membranes (in particular the mouth, throat and nose)

Does it interact with any other medicines? Yes. The following interactions are known:

- *Sedative effects*: Can be exacerbated if administered with clonazepam, chlordiazepoxide, diazepam, lorazepam, promethazine, zopiclone

Caution:

- Recommendation for regular ECGs
- Gradual withdrawal
- Symptoms of depression can occur

Drug name: Naltrexone - used for the prevention of relapse for individuals who have achieved abstinence for at least seven to ten days

UK brand names: Nalorex, Opizone

Average doses: Initial 25mg dose followed by 50mg daily dose, can be administered less frequently to support compliance. 350mg maximum weekly

What form does it come in? Tablet

Common side effects: Nausea and vomiting, diarrhoea, constipation, stomach cramp, dizziness, headaches, feeling thirsty, loss of appetite, poor sleep, **lethargy**, excessive energy, irritability, labile mood, skin rash, chills, urine retention, sweating, sexual dysfunction

Does it interact with other medicines? Yes. The following interactions are known:

- *Other medications*: Can precipitate withdrawal symptoms and prevent the medication from working if used with: buprenorphine, chlorpheniramine, methadone

Caution:

- Long-term use can cause serious implications and disruption for the sexual function of males and females, causing such side effects as impotence and infertility
- Repeated use is associated with dependence both psychologically and physically
- Recommendation for regular ECGs

CANNABIS

As the most widely used drug in the UK, with about 10 per cent of users classed as addicted (NHS, 2020a), cannabis is an illicit drug that a large proportion of those living with mental illness use. It is also a drug that has been extensively researched over the last ten years, particularly in relation to its impact on the mental health of individuals. The findings suggest a severe impact on individuals who are genetically vulnerable and suggest that these individuals may be more likely to develop a long and enduring psychotic illness if using cannabis (Royal College of Psychiatrists, 2014).

Cannabis withdrawal

Cannabis is a drug that can be detected by urine drug screen (UDS) for a period of about 28 days. The withdrawal effects are often psychological and can be as follows:

- Insomnia
- Irritability
- Low mood
- Anxiety
- Paranoia
- Restlessness
- Headaches
- Weight gain or loss.

How we can support the service user

There are no specific medicines available for service users to support them when withdrawing from cannabis use. It is essential to offer emotional support and monitor any changes in their physical health that could need treating.

We can also offer PRN medications such as sleep aids where appropriate but we need to ensure that we are mindful of previous drug history and dependence issues.

Smoking cannabis with tobacco is one of the most common methods of usage. It could therefore be beneficial to explore NRT options.

COCAINE

There are over a million regular cocaine users in the UK. It is a widely available drug that can be smoked, snorted and in some cases individuals inject it.

Cocaine is associated with a high risk of addiction due to the very strong psychological dependence that it can cause (NHS, 2020b). It can give individuals a greater sense of confidence and can create a sense of euphoria and sometimes even of grandiosity: these effects can encourage people to use it frequently, particularly if they struggle with social situations or self-validation. Its use is most commonly linked to mental health conditions such as anxiety and low mood.

The physical effects that cocaine use can have on individuals include increased heart rate, erosion of the nasal membrane(s) and risk of exposure to needle-sharing infection(s).

Signs and symptoms of cocaine withdrawal

Cocaine is a drug that can be detected by UDS for about 72 hours. Key withdrawal symptoms include:

- Irritability
- Low mood
- Fatigue
- Sore nose
- Heart palpitation.

How we can support the service user

There are no specific medicines available for service users to support them when withdrawing from cocaine use; however, it is essential to offer emotional support and monitor any changes in their physical health that could require treatment. We can also use pharmacological interventions to treat some of the symptoms being experienced, ensuring that we are mindful of previous drug history and dependence risk.

AMPHETAMINE-TYPE STIMULANTS

Common drugs in this group are speed, crystal meth, ephedrine and MDMA/ecstasy.

This group of drugs is most commonly associated with individuals who want to be more alert and energised, and are often used to stay awake for long periods of time. The deprivation of not sleeping or having any rest can have severe implications for the mental health of users. Agitated mood and panic attacks are very common, and on occasions psychotic episodes can be triggered. It is common for individuals to be admitted to services due to drug-induced psychosis associated with this group. In these cases, **psychotropic** medications are avoided until the influence of the drug has passed and an accurate assessment can be made.

Signs and symptoms of amphetamine withdrawal

Amphetamine-type stimulants can be detected by UDS for a period of about 72 hours. Common withdrawal symptoms include:

- Irritability
- Low mood
- Sore mouth
- Heart palpitation
- Raised body temperature.

How can we support the service user?

There are no specific medicines available for service users to support them when withdrawing from amphetamine type stimulants. However, it is essential to offer emotional support and monitor any changes in their physical health that could need treating, whilst treating for the side effects and offering support.

DEPENDENCE ON PRESCRIPTION MEDICATIONS

When we discuss substance abuse, it is important to acknowledge that medications that are often prescribed and medicines that are available over the counter can also create dependence.

The following prescription medications can be associated with substance abuse and dependence:

- Benzodiazepines
- Tramadol
- Codeine
- Morphine
- Dihydrocodeine
- Methadone
- Buprenorphine

- Promethazine
- Zopiclone.

Due to the accessibility of these medications, it can be extremely easy for individuals to become dependent and for healthcare professionals to be unaware of this. Service users in this situation may need to be prescribed a reduction programme to support them in breaking the cycle of dependence that has been created in the safest way clinically possible.

SUPPORTING RECOVERY FROM DRUG AND ALCOHOL DEPENDENCE IN PREGNANT WOMEN AND BREASTFEEDING MOTHERS

All the substances discussed in this chapter are associated with high risks for this client group, the most common being:

- Neonatal abnormalities
- Fetal dependence
- Stillbirth
- Premature birth
- Low birth weight
- Delayed brain development
- Secretion of drugs through breast milk.

It is essential to familiarise yourself with specific drug-related risks for care and treatment planning, and to educate the service user about these risks in order to help inform their decision-making.

CONSIDERATIONS FOR DIFFERENT AGE GROUPS

Substance misuse can affect people of all ages. Current data (Public Health England, 2019) shows an increase in those over 40, especially those using opiates and alcohol. This data suggests that we are seeing an ageing core group of people who have particularly high levels of substance misuse levels, with lower numbers of young people first developing such needs (especially for opiates and alcohol). There was an epidemic of increased heroin use in the 1980s and 1990s, and this group of people is now over 40. In 2017 to 2018, the data shows that of people with an opiate addiction, 69 per cent said they first used heroin before 2001 and only 9 per cent first used heroin since 2011.

This chapter will not give particular recommendations and guidelines for treating older people and younger people as such treatment is highly specialist and based on many factors. There should be a strong focus on psychosocial and psychological interventions at all ages (NICE, 2012).

Both older people (Kuerbis et al., 2014) and younger people (Mirza and Mirza, 2008) are at an increased risk of complications when they take any mood-altering substances, and there is a particular risk with older adults that any perceived tolerance levels they have developed when younger may change as they age, placing them more at risk of resulting accidents and harm. With young people, the focus on treatment should be around breaking the cycle and developing other, healthy coping mechanisms, to prevent the substance use continuing into adult life.

LEARNING FROM A CASE STUDY: TEST YOUR KNOWLEDGE

Leo is 39 years old and has a stressful job working in finance in Central London. His job often means he has to work late in the evenings, visiting restaurants and bars with potential clients in order to try to obtain business. Leo has just been informally admitted to the acute inpatient ward after being found sobbing inconsolably in the street. When an off-duty policeman asked him if he was OK, Leo said he wanted to 'end it all'.

During Leo's initial assessment on the ward, he states that he struggles with his self-esteem and that he has been using cocaine in order to help him feel more confident when he is socialising with clients:

1   You decide to do a UDS to see if cocaine is present in Leo's system. How long does cocaine remain in the system, and will it show up on a UDS?
2   Leo asks you if there are any risks of withdrawal from cocaine. What do you advise?

Whilst talking to Leo, he also tells you that he has been using alcohol. He says that he has been drinking two bottles of wine a night, every day of the week.

3   What are your worries?
4   What immediate nursing care do you need to put into place for Leo?
5   What type of medicine is most likely to be prescribed to support Leo whilst he is withdrawing from alcohol?

IF I REMEMBER 5 THINGS FROM THIS CHAPTER ...

1   Alcohol and/or substance abuse are often comorbid with mental health problems, and screening of drug and alcohol use should occur for all people coming into contact with mental health services.
2   People will have different reasons for using substances, and an individualised assessment is essential in order to develop person-centred treatment plans.
3   The concept of recovery is at the heart of all treatment for alcohol and substance abuse.
4   All service users undergoing withdrawal from alcohol and/or substances will need close physical monitoring and extensive emotional support.
5   When treating opiate withdrawal with medicines, substitution regimes are required. These are complex, and the medicines used are controlled drugs. Controlled drugs procedures must be followed at all times.

ANSWERS TO THE CASE STUDY QUESTIONS

1   Cocaine will remain in the system and show in a UDS for up to 72 hours following last use.
2   You advise Leo that there are some common withdrawal symptoms from cocaine. These include irritability, low mood, fatigue, sore nose and heart palpitations. You advise Leo that the team will be there to support him through these.
3   You should be worried about the withdrawal effects of alcohol. There are both physical and psychological withdrawal effects and these can be serious. They can include seizures and hallucinations.
4   Leo needs an urgent medical review – a full physical health assessment, and frequent physical monitoring. He will also need a high level of emotional support.
5   Benzodiazepines are the most commonly prescribed type of medicine to help with alcohol withdrawal.

REFERENCES AND RECOMMENDED READING

Abramson, A. (2021) 'Substance use during the pandemic', *American Psychological Association*, 52 (2), 22.

Action on Smoking and Health (ASH) (2016) 'High rates of smoking among people with serious mental health conditions'. Available at: https://ash. org.uk/media-and-news/press-releases-media-and-news/high-rates-of-smoking-among-people-with-serious-mental-health-conditions (accessed 25 June 2017).

Action on Smoking and Health (ASH) (2017) Fact sheets. Available at: https://ash.org.uk/fact-sheets (accessed 19 June 2017).

Department of Health (DH) (2016) UK Chief Medical Officers' Low Risk Drinking Guidelines. Available at: www.gov.uk/government/uploads/ system/uploads/attachment_data/file/545937/UK_CMOs__report.pdf (accessed 19 June 2017).

Department of Health (DH) (England) and the devolved administrations (2007) *Drug Misuse and Dependence: UK Guidelines on Clinical Management.* London: Department of Health (England), the Scottish Government, Welsh Assembly Government and Northern Ireland Executive. Available at: https://webarchive.nationalarchives.gov.uk/ukgwa/20170807160623/ http://www.nta.nhs.uk/uploads/clinical_guidelines_2007.pdf (last accessed 30 September 2021).

Di Chiara, G., Tanda, G., Cadoni, C., et al. (1998) 'Homologies and differences in the action of drugs of abuse and a conventional reinforcer (food) on dopamine transmission: An interpretive framework of the mechanism of drug dependence', *Advances in Pharmacology*, 42: 983–7.

DiClemente, C. (2007) 'The transtheoretical model of intentional behaviour change', *Drugs and Alcohol Today*, 7 (1): 29–33.

FRANK (n.d.) 'Drugs A–Z'. Available at: www.talktofrank.com (last accessed 30 September 2021).

Joint Formulary Committee (2017) *British National Formulary*, 73rd edn. London: British Medical Association (BMA) and Pharmaceutical Press.

Kuerbis, A., Sacco, P., Blazer, D.G., et al. (2014) 'Substance abuse among older adults', *Clinical and Geriatric Medicine*, 30 (3): 629–54.

McManus, S., Meltzer, H., Brugha, T.S., et al. (eds) (2009) *Adult Psychiatric Morbidity in England, 2007: Results of a Household Survey*. London: NHS Information Centre for Health and Social Care.

Mental Health Taskforce Strategy to the NHS England (2016) *The Five Year Forward View for Mental Health*. Available at: www.england.nhs.uk/ wp-content/uploads/2016/02/Mental-Health-Taskforce-FYFV-final.pdf (accessed 19 June 2017).

Mirza, K. and Mirza, S. (2008) Adolescent substance misuse. *Psychiatry*, 7 (8): 357– 62.

National Institute on Drug Abuse (NIDA) (2016) 'Substance use in women: Substance use while pregnant and breastfeeding'. Bethesda, MD: NIDA, National Institutes of Health (NIH), US Department of Health and Human Services. Available at: www.drugabuse.gov/publications/research-reports/ substance-use-in-women/substance-use-while-pregnant-breastfeeding (accessed 29 June 2017).

NHS (2020a). Cannabis: The facts. Available online at www.nhs.uk/live-well/ healthy-body/cannabis-the-facts (accessed 4 November 2021).

NHS (2020b) Drug addiction: Getting Help. Available online at www.nhs.uk/ live-well/healthy-body/drug-addiction-getting-help/ (accessed 4 November 2021)

NHS (2021) 'Addiction: What is it?' Available at: www.nhs.uk/Livewell/ addiction/Pages/addictionwhatisit.aspx (accessed 4 November 2021).

NHS Digital (2020) 'Statistics on drug misuse, England 2020'. Available at: https://digital.nhs.uk/data-and-information/publications/statistical/ statistics-on-drug-misuse/2020 (accessed 5 July 2021).

NICE (2012) 'Quality standard: Drug use disorders in adults'. Available at www.nice.org.uk/guidance/qs23 (accessed 5 July 2021).

NICE (2013) 'Smoking: Acute, maternity and mental health services'. Public health guideline 48. Available at www.nice.org.uk/guidance/ph48 (accessed 30 September 2021).

Nursing & Midwifery Council (NMC) (2020) *The Code*. Available at: www. nmc.org.uk/standards/code/ (accessed 5 July 2021).

Preedy, V. (2016) *Neuropathy of Drug Addictions and Substance Misuse, Vol. 1: Foundations of Understanding Tobacco, Alcohol, Cannabinoids and Opioids*. London: Elsevier.

Prochaska, J. and DiClemente, C. (1984) *The Transtheoretical Approach: Towards a Systematic Eclectic Framework*. Homewood, IL: Dow Jones Irwin.

Public Health England (2016) Adult Substance Misuse Statistics from the National Drug Treatment Monitoring System (NDTMS). Available at: https://webarchive.nationalarchives.gov.uk/ ukgwa/20170807160623/http://www.nta.nhs.uk/uploads/adult-statistics- from-the-national-drug-treatment-monitoring-system-2015-2016[0].pdf (accessed 30 September 2021).

Public Health England (2019) 'Adult substance misuse treatment statistics 2018 to 2019: report'. Available at: www.gov.uk/government/statistics/ substance-misuse-treatment-for-adults-statistics-2018-to-2019/adult- substance-misuse-treatment-statistics-2018-to-2019-report (accessed 5 July 2021).

Repper, J. and Perkins, R. (2003) *Social Inclusion and Recovery: A Model for Mental Health Practice*. London: Baillière Tindall.

Resnicow, K. and McMaster, F. (2012) 'Motivational interviewing: Moving from why to how with autonomy support', *International Journal of Behavioural Nutrition and Physical Activity*, 9: 19.

Royal College of Psychiatrists (2014) Cannabis. www.rcpsych.ac.uk.

Sattar, P. and Bhatia, S. (2003) 'Benzodiazepines for substance abusers', *Journal of Current Psychiatry*, 2 (5): 25–34.

Stead, L.F., Perera, R., Bullen, C., et al. (2012) 'Nicotine replacement therapy for smoking cessation', *Cochrane Database of Systematic Reviews*, 11 (14 November): CD000146. Doi: 10.1002/14651858.CD000146.pub4.

West, R. and Brown, J. (2013) *Theory of Addiction*, 2nd edn. London: Wiley Blackwell.

World Health Organization (WHO) (2012) *Management of Alcohol Withdrawal*. Available at: https://www.who.int/teams/mental-health-and-substance-use/treatment-care/mental-health-gap-action-programme/evidence-centre/alcohol-use-disorders/management-of-alcohol-withdrawal (accessed 28 June 2021).

5 ANTIPSYCHOTIC MEDICATION

LIZ HOLLAND

AFTER READING THIS CHAPTER, YOU WILL BE ABLE TO:

- Consider the needs of individuals who may take antipsychotic medication
- Have a basic awareness of how antipsychotic medications came about
- Hold a basic understanding of the different types of antipsychotic medications and how they work
- Consider the risks and benefits of different types of antipsychotic medication
- Apply basic knowledge around antipsychotic medications to clinical decision-making

---

WHY DO WE NEED ANTIPSYCHOTIC MEDICATION?

Psychosis has been named by some as the most severe and symbolic of the mental health diagnoses (Moncrieff, 2008) and has been poorly portrayed in the media; the impact of media coverage has led to some people seeing psychosis as 'dangerous'. This is not true: research from Mind (2020) states that you are more likely to get struck by lightning than you are to be attacked by someone with a mental health problem!

Psychotic illnesses are characterised by someone having a combination of positive symptoms (things that appear) such as hearing voices, seeing things that other people cannot see or believing that they have special powers, and negative symptoms (things that disappear) such as having very low energy levels, not feeling interested in things and not feeling motivated to look after oneself.

'Schizophrenia' and 'psychosis' are often used as interchangeable terms, but this is not correct. Psychosis refers to an experience in which a person experiences a temporary altered reality, whether that be through a loss of contact with reality or through a change in their belief system and perception. Some people can develop a one-off psychotic episode which may be linked to factors such as stress, exhaustion and drug use. Schizophrenia refers to lifelong illness in which a person suffers regular psychotic experiences and often needs long-term treatment to remain free of psychosis. Other mental health problems such as bipolar disorder and depression can include episodes of psychosis as part of their symptomatology.

John Nash, the famous mathematician, is one of the most well-known people to have suffered from schizophrenia, and in an interview live on CNN he summarised his experience of having a psychotic illness in the following way:

> I thought of the voices as ... something a little different from aliens. I thought of them more like angels ... It's really my subconscious talking, it was really that ... I know that now. (Nash, interview in 2002)

Up until the 1950s, people with enduring states of psychosis were considered incurable and 'mad' and were therefore largely confined to mental institutions and asylums, where treatments were limited. However, from the late 1950s, antipsychotic medicines began to come into use – although they were discovered by accident! The discovery of antipsychotic drug treatment coincided with the development of the dopamine theory of schizophrenia. This occurred through the discovery of something known as 'amphetamine psychosis'.

In the 1950s, it was noted that when people used amphetamine-based recreational drugs, the symptoms that they experienced were similar to those positive symptoms that were displayed by people with a psychotic illness – for example, seeing things that may not really be there or having abnormal sensory experiences. The way in which amphetamines work on the brain is that they cause a sudden rise in the levels of the neurotransmitter dopamine in the brain, and therefore a link between increased levels of dopamine and psychotic symptoms began to become established. In additional support of this dopamine hypothesis, it was noticed that when a drug called 'levodopa', which worked by increasing dopamine levels, was given to patients with Parkinson's disease, the patients showed side effects very similar to the positive symptoms of schizophrenia. This led to the simplistic deduction that the positive symptoms of schizophrenia must be caused by high levels of dopamine.

Therefore, in very simple terms, medicines that were known to reduce levels of dopamine in the brain were targeted for use in the treatment of psychotic illness, with chlorpromazine being the first of these drugs to be studied at length. As these medicines were found to have some beneficial effect on the reduction of psychotic symptoms, development continued, even though there remained very limited rationale and understanding. There is additionally much evidence that contradicts the dopamine theory of schizophrenia;

the neurochemical changes in the brain that occur after an antipsychotic drug is taken happen immediately and yet it can take days or weeks to see any behavioural changes take place. Neuroimaging studies suggest that the cause of psychotic illnesses is likely to be due to far more complex changes than just dopamine alone.

It is worth noting what Pies (2011) stated: 'In truth, the "chemical imbalance" notion was always a kind of urban legend – never a theory seriously propounded by well-informed psychiatrists'. However, there are, at this time, no other convincing biological theories around the causation of schizophrenia or rationale for antipsychotic medication that can be used as an alternative.

It should be noted that antipsychotic medication can be used as an emergency treatment to help calm down someone when they are particularly distressed or emotionally aroused. The use of antipsychotics for emergency treatment is covered in Chapter 6. This chapter focuses on antipsychotic medication given as regular treatment.

THE TWO DIFFERENT FAMILIES OF ANTIPSYCHOTIC MEDICATION AND THEIR SIDE EFFECTS

There are two different families of antipsychotic medicines, known as either the typical and the atypical medicines, or the first- and second-generation medicines. The older medicines are the ones known as 'typical' or 'first generation' and the newer medicines are known as 'atypical' or "second generation'. This book will use the terms 'typical' and 'atypical' to refer to the two different families moving forward. The typical and atypical antipsychotics have slightly different side effect profiles, although they also share some similarities in this area.

The typical antipsychotics were those that were first developed following the dopamine theory of the 1950s. As a result of this, the typical antipsychotics work predominantly on dopamine by blocking the action of dopamine in the brain. Although the typical antipsychotics were noted to have some effect on the positive symptoms of psychosis, they did not seem to affect the negative symptoms. The typical antipsychotics are particularly associated with severe neuromuscular side effects and movement disorders.

The atypical antipsychotics came along later, in the 1990s, and, although they still work by blocking dopamine, they do this to a lesser extent than the typical medications, and they also work on other neurotransmitters in the brain, such as serotonin. The atypical medicines have been noted to have some effect on negative as well as positive symptoms. Although the atypical medicines have developed less severe neuromuscular side effects than their older counterparts, they are associated with severe metabolic side effects such as rapid weight gain.

All the antipsychotic medications can cause severe side effects in individuals taking them, and these should be monitored and discussed; no one should have to put up with horrendous side effects!

The key side effects related to the typical antipsychotics include:

- Problems with breast tenderness and swelling in both men and women. Lactation may also occur. This is due to increases in a hormone called 'prolactin'
- Sexual side effects such as problems reaching climax, being able to get and/or sustain an erection and vaginal dryness
- Blood pressure changes, particularly postural hypotension, and associated feelings of dizziness
- Feeling tired and drowsy
- Feeling 'slowed down' in your thinking.

In addition to these are side effects known as 'extra-pyramidal side effects' (EPSEs). These are caused by the resulting lack of dopamine in the brain, and can look similar to the symptoms of Parkinson's disease. Each of these side effects has a fancy name. However, make sure that when you are discussing these with patients, you avoid the fancy names, and explain exactly what it is that you mean in order to avoid confusion:

- *Dystonia*: Sudden involuntary movements and muscle contractions. These can include abnormal mouth and tongue movements, and abnormal rolling of the eyes, known as 'oculogyric crisis'. These tend to appear early on, after starting a typical antipsychotic, usually within the first week.
- *Akathisia*: Feeling restless/inability to sit still.
- *Parkinsonism*: Feeling rigid or having very stiff muscles.
- *Bradykinesia*: Slowed-down movements.
- *Tardive dyskinesia*: Irregular, jerky movements. This can include abnormal movements or smacking of the lips, tongue and mouth. These tend to appear after someone has been taking typical antipsychotics for six months or longer, and can be hard to reverse once present.
- *Tremors*: Involuntary shaking of the hands, feet or limbs.

If patients do develop EPSEs, medicines known as **anticholinergic** drugs can be helpful at relieving some of these side effects, and, very basically, they affect the function of the central nervous system. Procyclidine is the one you are most likely to see being used in current practice.

For people suffering from akathisia, this can be debilitating and can need ongoing treatment, and this is one area that using anticholinergic medicines may be less effective. Instead, treatment options can include mirtazapine and benzodiazepines. Jethwa (2018) provides a helpful review in the treatment options in the article 'Pharmacological management of antipsychotic-induced akathisia: an update and treatment algorithm' (see reference at the end of the article to go on and read this), and they have produced the diagram below:

First-line management	Mirtazapine 15mg daily

Second-line management	Clonazepam 1mg daily

Third-line management	Propranolol 80mg daily, procyclidine 5mg daily (if Parkinsonian symptoms present)

- Treatment should be limited to 4 weeks for each agent before switching (if symptoms persist) or discontinuation (following symptomatic resolution)
- In addition to pharmacotherapy, patients should have regular risk assessments and structured psychosocial support and psychoeduction to help them manage their symptoms and aid medication adherence

Figure 5.1   Evidence-based treatment algorithm for the management of antipsychotic-induced akathisia. From Jethwa (2018).

Moving on to atypical antipsychotics, the key side effects include:

- Sexual, such as problems reaching climax, being able to get and/or sustain an erection and having vaginal dryness
- Feeling very sleepy
- Rapid weight gain. Such weight gain risks have also led to a link between atypical antipsychotics and the development of type 2 diabetes
- Blood pressure changes, particularly postural hypotension, and associated feelings of dizziness
- Constipation
- Having a dry mouth
- Blurred vision.

All of the antipsychotic medications have the potential to affect the rhythm of the heart, alongside all of the above. This will be discussed in more detail later in the chapter, together with how this should be managed by nursing staff. You should note that all of the above side effects can be incredibly unpleasant for the person experiencing them, and this may be enough to cause the person to stop taking their medication, which is why it is really important that these are discussed openly. More seriously, if health issues such as blood pressure changes, diabetes and constipation are not identified and treated early, then they can lead to severe illness and even death. Overall, it is suggested that as doses of medication increase, so, too, do the risks of developing side effects.

If you are working with a person who is experiencing side effects, it is so important that you start the conversation, and ask people about the impact that the side effects are having on their day-to-day life. The GASS tool in the box below can be incredibly helpful with this. If side effects are severe and/or causing the person distress, it is important to think about whether the dose can be quickly reduced, or the medication should be stopped and an alternative tried.

GO FURTHER ...

A simple side effect questionnaire or tool can be really helpful in starting a conversation with patients around antipsychotic medication and side effects. A really good one to look at is the Glasgow Antipsychotic Side-Effect Scale (GASS), developed by Waddell and Taylor (2008).

DEPOT MEDICATION

Some types of antipsychotic medication are available as long-acting depot injections rather than as an oral treatment. These injections can be used for people who make a personal choice to have an injection rather than take daily tablets, or for people for whom there may be concerns around compliance with regular oral medication.

The antipsychotic medicines that are given through an injection are fundamentally the same drug as their oral equivalent, and therefore the side effects remain the same. The medications are slow release, which means that a small amount of the medication is released daily from the muscle in which the injection into the blood stream is given. The injections are given on a regular basis, usually at one- to four-week intervals.

All **depot medications** are given as **IM (intramuscular) injections**, and the most popular injection site is currently the **dorsogluteal** area. A growing number of injections are now being developed for the deltoid site in order to allow patient choice and increased dignity, and the **ventrogluteal** site is also becoming a more popular alternative.

When a decision is made that someone is going to start on a depot medication, it is usual practice that the person will be given a very small amount of the medicine as an injection. This is called a 'test dose'. The person is then assessed for up to seven days following this in order to ensure that they have no severe side effects or reactions, before a bigger dose is given. If possible, it may also be a good idea to start the person on the oral equivalent of the planned depot medication so as to allow for an assessment of side effects, tolerance and response before moving to the injectable form.

When you administer a depot medication to a patient, it is really important to reassure them because, for some people, having an injection can be an anxious and stressful experience. You should always ensure that you are aware of which injection site you should be using, and also whether it is the left or right side that had the last injection; you should alternate your choice each time so as to ensure that the injection site does not become sore.

All depot injections should be given using the Z-tracking technique and following the principles of asepsis. All injectable medications should be prepared by the person giving the injection, and a second registered nurse should independently check the injection, before administration, once it is prepared in order to ensure that everything is correct.

Table 5.1 shows the medicines you may come across that can be given as depot medications.

Table 5.1 Antipsychotic depot medications

Medicine name	UK brand name	UK maximum dose	Typical frequency of injections	Current recommended injection site	Typical or atypical antipsychotic?
Haloperidol decanoate	Haldol	300mg	2-4 weekly	Dorsogluteal	Typical
Zuclopenthixol decanoate	Clopixol	600mg	1-4 weekly	Dorsogluteal	Typical
Pipotiazine palmitate	Piportil	200mg	4 weekly	Dorsogluteal	Typical
Fluphenazine decanoate	Modecate	100mg	2-5 weekly	Dorsogluteal	Typical

(Continued)

Table 5.1   (Continued)

Medicine name	UK brand name	UK maximum dose	Typical frequency of injections	Current recommended injection site	Typical or atypical antipsychotic?
Flupentixol decanoate	Depixol	400mg	2-4 weekly	Dorsogluteal	Typical
Olanzapine	ZypAdhera	405mg	2 or 4 weekly	Dorsogluteal	Atypical
Risperidone	Risperdal Consta	50mg	2 weekly	Deltoid	Atypical
Paliperidone	Xeplion	150mg	4 weekly	Deltoid	Atypical
Aripiprazole	Abilify Maintena	400mg	Monthly	Dorsogluteal	Atypical

KEY ISSUES TO BE AWARE OF WITH ANTIPSYCHOTIC MEDICATION AND RECOMMENDATIONS FOR NURSING CARE

As discussed above, the side effects of both families of antipsychotic medications can be serious and severe. Alongside regular conversations around side effects, there are some other elements of care that all nursing staff should provide to patients who are taking antipsychotic medications.

All the antipsychotic medications, but particularly the atypicals, can cause constipation. If constipation is not treated, it can lead to bowel blockages, blood poisoning and death. It is therefore really important to know about the bowel habits of your patients: yes, there is no need to be embarrassed, you need to open a conversation and get talking about poo! It is a good idea to encourage patients who take clozapine to keep a stool chart or log so that signs of constipation can be identified early. You should talk patients through the signs and symptoms of constipation using a tool such as the Bristol Stool Chart and also encourage people to eat lots of fruit, vegetables and complex carbohydrates to maximise their fibre intake, as well as drink plenty of fluids and stay physically active, as this stimulates the bowel.

The rapid weight gain associated with antipsychotic medication can be incredibly distressing, and research from Tschoner et al. (2007) states that the average person taking antipsychotic medication will experience a long-term weight increase of at least 25 per cent. Allison et al. (2009) suggest that, for atypical drugs, weight gain can be over 4 kg in just the first 10 weeks. Therefore, it is really important that we regularly monitor the weight of patients taking antipsychotic medication and provide health and lifestyle advice.

These conversations can be hard but are extremely important. It is also really important to consider the other health risks that may occur if someone becomes overweight, such as diabetes and heart disease, and to provide regular health screening for these.

Looking after the heart is particularly important in people who are on antipsychotic medications as, alongside the increased risk of being overweight, these medicines can interfere with the electrical rhythm of the heart, especially the QTc interval. Changes in the electrical rhythm of the heart can lead to changes in blood pressure and a very high or low heart rate. There are also, sadly, links between antipsychotic medicines and sudden arrhythmic death syndrome (SADS); these risks are particularly high for the typical antipsychotics (Glassman and Bigger, 2001). Due to the high risk of cardiac complications, all patients who are taking an antipsychotic should have an ECG prior to starting on the medication and before any dose changes. An ECG should then be carried out on a regular one- to three-month basis whilst the person continues taking antipsychotic medication. The risk of complications becomes higher if the person is on a higher dose of medication, and so people taking high doses may need more frequent monitoring.

In addition to an ECG, there are other health checks that must be conducted before starting on antipsychotic medication. These are:

- A physical examination, including pulse, blood pressure, respiration rate, temperature, height, weight, waist measurement, blood glucose, diet, activity levels and an assessment for any signs of movement disorder
- Blood tests to look at cholesterol levels, prolactin levels, haemoglobin and blood sugar levels

Alongside regular ECGs, patients who are stable on antipsychotic medication should have a full physical health check at least once every 12 months.

Another reason for which the above health checks are so important for people on antipsychotic medications is the risk of 'metabolic syndrome'. Metabolic syndrome refers to a group of risk factors which, when together, greatly increase a person's risk of heart disease and type 2 diabetes. Collins et al. (2013) define the key features of metabolic syndrome as: insulin resistance, elevated insulin levels in the blood, visceral obesity, glucose intolerance, elevated cholesterol levels and central obesity. Clinically, patients at risk of metabolic syndrome will likely have: a high body mass index (BMI), elevated blood pressure, elevated blood glucose and a waist measurement of 101.6+ cm (40+ inches) in men and 93.98+ cm (37+ inches) in women (Collins et al., 2013). Research has suggested that people taking antipsychotic medication are at increased risk of acquiring metabolic syndrome, and this is likely to be due to more than just possible increased body weight: 25 per cent of patients who develop metabolic syndrome on antipsychotics do not show any increased body weight, which suggests that the drugs are having a direct effect on the metabolic system in some way (Collins et al., 2013). The atypicals have a stronger link with metabolic syndrome than the typicals, with olanzapine and clozapine being found to be the 'worst offenders'.

The final thing to be aware of is the link between antipsychotic medications and blood disorders. Antipsychotic medications affect the bone marrow, and this can lead to a decrease in the levels of white blood cells. Clozapine is particularly high risk in relation to this, but it can occur with any antipsychotic medication. In rare cases, the body can suddenly cease producing any white blood cells, leading to a crisis known as neuroleptic malignant syndrome (NMS). The **mortality** rate for NMS is 10–15 per cent and so it is extremely important that it is identified and treated as quickly as possible. Clinically, patients with NMS may show a sudden increased temperature, experience initial muscle pain, stiffness and rigidity, an irregular and fast pulse, high or low blood pressure, excessive sweating, a high respiration state and severe confusion. Any patient on antipsychotics with any of these symptoms needs an urgent blood test: high levels of creatine phosphate are the key indicator to confirm a diagnosis of NMS. It is more likely to occur at the start of new antipsychotic treatment but can happen at any time. In cases of NMS or likely NMS, all antipsychotic medication must be ceased immediately, and must be reintroduced very cautiously and slowly once the person has received clinical treatment for the symptoms of NMS and is physically well again.

WORKING WITH CLOZAPINE

Clozapine is one of the newer antipsychotic oral medications, classed as an atypical, and is used for people who have not responded to other types of psychiatric medication. The prescribing guidance for clozapine is that the person must have previously taken at least two other antipsychotic medications for a reasonable amount of time, with at least one of them being atypical, without a response. Around 30–60 per cent of patients who have not responded to other medicines will show a response to clozapine (Dixon and Dada, 2014).

Although clozapine can be effective in some cases, the decision to take clozapine should not be taken lightly because it can have very severe side effects. There is a risk of blood disorders and cardiac problems, and these are discussed in more detail below.

Due to the risks of the side effects, there are very specific rules in place that you need to be aware of as a nurse when supporting people who are on clozapine, including the following key issues.

Clozapine bloods

All patients on clozapine need regular blood monitoring. A full set of bloods, including a white blood cell count, should be done within ten days prior to starting the clozapine treatment. An ECG must always be completed.

For the first 18 weeks of treatment, a blood test is needed every week. After this, blood tests can be done fortnightly for the rest of the first year. After this first year, bloods can be done on a four-weekly basis as long as there are no identified problems or changes to dose.

The blood tests are checking the clozapine level in the blood and the white blood cell count. The reason for this is that clozapine can cause a sudden drop in neutrophils, which are a type of white blood cell. Approximately 2 per cent of patients taking clozapine will experience a small fall in their neutrophil level (neutropenia) and less than 1 per cent of patients taking clozapine will experience a large fall in their neutrophil level (agranulocytosis; see Dixon and Dada, 2014).

Agranulocytosis and neutropenia are uncommon and can occur at any time but are most common within the first 18 weeks of treatment.

A prescription for clozapine cannot be given without the blood test results: the prescription will only be made if the results of the blood test are OK, and the prescription will only provide enough medication until the date of the next blood test.

Clozapine blood results will come back as 'green', 'amber' or 'red':

Green result: White cell count > 3.0, neutrophil count > 1.5

This means that the blood test is normal and so the planned treatment with clozapine can continue.

Amber result: White cell count 2.5–3, neutrophil count 1.0–1.5

This means that the blood test is within the required range but is moving towards an area of concern and needs close monitoring. Treatment can continue, but another blood test may need to be done sooner than planned in order to check that everything is OK.

Red result: white cell count < 2.5, neutrophil count < 1.0

This means that the person has a low number of white blood cells. The blood monitoring experts will contact the person's doctor straight away. Another blood test should be arranged straight away in order to confirm the result of the first test. Treatment will be stopped immediately until the result is available. If the number of white cells in the blood is confirmed to be low, clozapine will need to be stopped and the person will require close physical monitoring until the white blood cell count returns to normal.

If clozapine is stopped, an alternative treatment for the person needs to be considered, and the risk of relapse also needs to be acknowledged and a plan for this should be created with the person.

When interpreting blood results, you should be aware of a person's ethnic background as people of an African or African Carribean background may have a naturally lower level of white blood cells, and this is perfectly normal for them.

Clozapine titration and doses

An ECG and full set of bloods must be taken prior to the commencement of clozapine treatment. Clozapine is usually started with a dose of 12.5mg once or twice on the first day, and this is then followed by one or two 25mg tablets on the second day. Blood pressure, pulse, temperature and respiration rate must be checked and recorded before the medication can be given (you need to withhold the medication and discuss with a doctor if the patient's heart rate is above 110 beats per minute (bpm), as this is a sign that the clozapine is affecting the patient's cardiac system and is causing tachycardia).

If the patient appears to tolerate the medication well, then the daily dose may be increased slowly in increments of 25mg to 50mg until a dose of up to 300mg/day is achieved. This normally takes two to three weeks. After this, if required, the daily dose may be further increased in increments of 50mg to 100mg at half-weekly or, preferably, weekly intervals.

In most patients, a dose of 300–450mg/day (given in divided doses) is found to be the optimum dose. Some patients may be treated with lower doses, and some patients may require doses of up to 600mg/day. The total daily dose may be divided unevenly, with the larger portion being taken at bedtime, as larger doses can cause the patient to become drowsy.

Rarely, some patients may require a dose in excess of 600mg daily. The dose can be increased in 100mg increments up to a maximum of 900mg daily. However, doses of over 450mg are more likely to lead to adverse reactions, in particular, seizures.

Stopping and then restarting clozapine

For any patient who has missed more than two days of clozapine treatment, the medication needs to be stopped. The usual dose cannot be given and retitration is required. Treatment should be reinitiated with 12.5mg (half a 25mg tablet) given once or twice on the first day. If this dose is well tolerated, it may be feasible to titrate the dose back to the original dose more quickly than when initially starting treatment. Weekly bloods will be needed for a short time.

Other important information

Changing the number of cigarettes smoked or the amount of caffeine consumed can affect the amount of clozapine in the blood. Therefore, it is important that you know the smoking and drinking habits of patients before they commence treatment, and that these are monitored and discussed regularly. Patients should not change their smoking habits or caffeine intake without meeting with a healthcare professional.

Going on holiday can be difficult for people who take clozapine, and the guidance is that holidays away from people's local area are not advisable, and they need to be well planned if they do happen.

If the period of time that the person is going away for means that they will miss a blood-monitoring appointment, then special arrangements need to be made by a doctor or nurse. It is also important that the person and anyone travelling with them knows what to do if the person on clozapine develops signs of an infection, such as raised temperature and flu-like symptoms which can suggest a decrease in the white blood cell count. If there is any concern that a person on clozapine has developed an infection whilst on holiday, then medical advice must be obtained immediately.

If the person is staying in the UK, then their consultant should make sure that blood-monitoring requirements are met during the time of the holiday. If a blood test is due during the holiday, the treating psychiatrist should arrange for the test to be done with a psychiatrist at the person's holiday destination. This stand-in psychiatrist will:

- Take any routine blood samples and send them to the laboratory
- Be notified of the blood test result
- Authorise the supply of clozapine tablets if the blood test is OK
- Be the emergency contact for the person and the laboratory.

If the person wishes to go abroad, then before the person travels their psychiatrist will need to set up an emergency contact number so that the treatment team can be reached at any time. They should also check that there were no concerns with the previous blood test results and notify the laboratory of the holiday plans.

THE MEDICINES LIST

This list will look at the most commonly used antipsychotic medicines in UK mental health services, and these medicines will be split into the categories of typical and atypical medications. The side effect profiles for each medication have already been discussed, but any specific side effects for each medication will be highlighted here. The chemical name and UK brand name of each drug will be given, the average doses and any important contraindications to be aware of. This is not an exhaustive list of all the antipsychotic medications. You can download a list of all the antipsychotics and their properties that are currently being used in the UK at: www.mind.org.uk/information-support/drugs-and-treatments/antipsychotics-a-z/overview/?o=38598. Remember, as a nurse, you are responsible for knowing and understanding each medicine you dispense and administer to a patient (NMC, 2015). Clozapine and depot-only medications are not covered in this section as they have already been discussed.

The typical antipsychotics

Drug name: **Chlorpromazine**

UK brand names: Largactil

Average doses:

- Oral: 75–300mg daily
- Suppository: 100mg daily

What form does it come in? Tablet, liquid, solution for emergency injection, suppository

Does it interact with any other medicines? Yes. The following interactions are known:

- *Propranolol:* If you take propranolol and chlorpromazine together, blood levels of both drugs can increase
- *Haloperidol:* Chlorpromazine can increase the blood levels of haloperidol if they are taken together

Caution:

- Chlorpromazine can increase skin sensitivity to sunlight

Drug name: Haloperidol

UK brand names: Dozic, Haldol, Haldol decanoate (depot), Serenace

Average doses:

- *Depot*: 300mg every four weeks
- *Oral:* 1-3mg three times daily
- *IM injection*: 2-5mg daily

What form does it come in? Tablet, capsule, liquid, emergency injection, depot injection

Does it interact with any other medicines? Yes. The following interactions are known:

- *Carbamazepine:* Carbamazepine can reduce the blood level of haloperidol
- *Chlorpromazine:* If chlorpromazine and haloperidol are taken together, the blood levels of haloperidol may increase
- *Clozapine:* Clozapine and haloperidol depot should not be given together as there is a risk of blood disorder, and treatment cannot be stopped quickly should this occur
- *Fluoxetine:* If fluoxetine and haloperidol are taken together, the blood levels of haloperidol may increase
- *Fluvoxamine:* If fluvoxamine and haloperidol are taken together, the blood levels of haloperidol may increase
- *Lithium:* Taking lithium and haloperidol together increases risk of NMS
- *SSRI antidepressants:* If taken with haloperidol, these can lead to an increased risk of serious disturbances of heart rhythm
- *Sulpiride:* If taken with haloperidol, there is an increased risk of irregular heartbeat

(Continued)

- *Tricyclic antidepressants:* If taken with haloperidol, these can lead to an increased risk of serious disturbances of heart rhythm
- *Venlafaxine:* If venlafaxine and haloperidol are taken together, the blood levels of haloperidol may increase

Caution:

- Can cause excessive drowsiness, therefore consciousness level should be monitored.

Drug name: **Sulpiride**

UK brand names: Dolmatil, Sulpor

Average doses: 400-800mg daily

What form does it come in? Tablet and liquid

Does it interact with any other medicines? Yes. The following interactions are known:

- *Haloperidol*: If haloperidol and sulpiride are taken together, there is increased risk of dangerous disturbances of heart rhythm
- *Lithium*: Taking lithium and sulpiride together can lead to an increased risk of neuromuscular side effects
- *Pimozide*: Taking pimozide and sulpiride together can cause an increased risk of change to the heart's rhythm
- *Tricyclic antidepressant*: If taken with sulpiride, this can lead to an increased risk of serious disturbances to the heart rhythm

---

Drug name: **Trifluoperazine**

UK brand names: Stelazine

Average doses: 10-15mg daily

What form does it come in? Tablet and liquid

Does it interact with any other medicines? Yes. The following interactions are known:

- *Lithium*: If taken together with trifluoperazine, blood levels of the trifluoperazine may reduce. Additionally, there is an increased risk of movement disorders and a possible risk of sleepwalking

Caution:

- Linked to cases of NMS and tardive dyskinesia
- Neuromuscular side effects are more likely at doses over 6mg

The atypical antipsychotics

Drug name: **Aripiprazole**

UK brand names: Abilify, Abilify Maintena (depot)

Average doses:

- For schizophrenia: 10-15mg
- For mania: 15mg
- Depot injection: 400mg per month
- Total recommended daily maximum in all forms: 30mg

What form does it come in? Tablet, liquid, solution for emergency injection and depot injection

Does it interact with any other medicines? Yes. The following interactions are known:

- *Carbamazepine*: Carbamazepine can decrease the efficacy of aripiprazole
- *Lorazepam*: If lorazepam and aripiprazole are taken together, there is an increased risk of low blood pressure
- *SSRI and SNRI antidepressants*: There is an increased risk of serotonin syndrome if these are taken alongside aripiprazole
- *St John's wort*: St John's wort can decrease the efficacy of aripiprazole

Caution:

- May increase the effects of alcohol

(Continued)

- If starting on aripiprazole depot, the person should not start the depot without having been on the tablets first; and when they start on the depot, they should continue with tablets for the first two weeks

Drug name: Olanzapine

UK brand names: Zalasta, Zyprexa, ZypAdhera (depot)

Average doses:

- For schizophrenia and bipolar disorder: 5–10mg
- For a manic episode: 15mg
- Depot injection: 150mg every two weeks or 300mg every four weeks
- Total recommended daily maximum in all forms: 20mg

What form does it come in? Tablet, orodispersible tablet, solution for emergency injection and depot injection

Does it interact with any other medicines? Yes. The following interactions are known:

- *Benzodiazepines given by IM*: If given together, then there is an increased risk of low blood pressure, low pulse and low respiration rate
- *Carbamazepine*: Carbamazepine can reduce the blood level of olanzapine
- *Fluvoxamine*: Fluvoxamine can increase plasma levels of olanzapine
- *Lithium*: Taking olanzapine alongside lithium increases the risk of lithium toxicity
- *Valproate*: Taking valproate alongside olanzapine can increase the risk of a reduced white blood cell count

Caution:

- Particularly linked with increased and rapid weight gain

Drug name: Quetiapine

UK brand names: Atrolak, Biquelle, Ebesque, Seroquel, Tenprolide, Zaluron

Average doses:

- For schizophrenia: 300-450mg
- For mania: 200-800mg
- For depression in bipolar: 300mg
- For prevention of mania and depression in bipolar: 300-800mg

What form does it come in? Tablet only

Does it interact with any other medicines? Yes. The following interactions are known:

- *Carbamazepine*: Carbamazepine can reduce the blood level of quetiapine
- *Lithium*: If taken together, there are increased risks of sleepiness, weight gain and neuromuscular side effects

Caution:

- Medicine may need to be taken at different times of the day, depending on the treatment plan
- Patients should not consume grapefruit juice whilst on quetiapine, as this can increase quetiapine blood levels

Drug name: Risperidone

UK brand names: Risperdal, Risperdal Consta (depot)

Average daily dose:

- For psychoses: 4-6mg
- For mania: 1-6mg
- Depot injection: 25mg every two weeks
- Total recommended daily maximum taken orally: 16mg
- Total recommended maximum for depot: 50mg every two weeks

What form does it come in? Tablet, liquid and depot injection

(Continued)

Does it interact with any other medicines? Yes. The following interactions are known:

- *Carbamazepine*: Carbamazepine can reduce the blood level of risperidone
- *Clozapine*: Clozapine and risperidone depot should not be given together as there is a risk of blood disorder, and treatment could not be stopped quickly should this occur
- *Fluoxetine*: If fluoxetine and risperidone are taken together, the blood levels of risperidone may increase
- *Lithium*: Taking lithium and risperidone together increases the risk of NMS
- *Paroxetine*: Paroxetine is known to increase the adverse effects of risperidone
- *Tricyclic antidepressants*: If taken with risperidone, these can lead to an increased risk of serious disturbances of the heart rhythm

Caution:

- If starting on the risperidone depot, you should not be given the depot injection unless you have already been on the tablets or liquid
- Risperidone should not be given to people with dementia because it increases the risk of stroke

Drug name: Amisulpride

UK brand names: Solian

Average doses:

- For acute psychotic episodes: 400-800mg
- To target negative symptoms: 50-300mg

What form does it come in? Tablet and liquid

Does it interact with any other medicines? Yes. The following interactions are known:

- *Benzodiazepines*: Taking amisulpride and benzodiazepines together can increase sedative effects

Caution:

- May increase the effects of alcohol

ANTIPSYCHOTICS IN PREGNANT WOMEN AND BREASTFEEDING MOTHERS

The use of antipsychotic medication in new and expectant mothers remains a very under-researched area, and there is only limited information available. Due to the paucity of such information, Green et al. (2013) state that there is no psychiatric medication that is completely safe for use in pregnancy and recommend that best practice is to avoid all psychotropic drugs during pregnancy. However, if the mother is at risk of deteriorating or relapsing should she come off her antipsychotic medication, then it may be considered best that she remains on her medication. Any new or expectant mother should receive advice and support from specialist perinatal mental health services as well as her mental health nurse and her midwife.

Overall, the first trimester is considered to be the riskiest time in pregnancy to take any psychiatric medication, and there is some evidence that antipsychotic medication can cause problems with organ development in the unborn baby if taken during this time. The second trimester seems to be the lowest risk, and the third trimester is linked with withdrawal symptoms in the baby when it is born, alongside temporary muscle disorders. It is recommended that any expectant mother taking antipsychotic medication should take folic acid throughout the pregnancy as this can help to reduce the risk of the development of birth defects (Babu et al., 2015).

Another problem with research into antipsychotic drug use in pregnancy is highlighted by Robakis and Williams (2013), who say that it is very hard to distinguish between what is the side effect of the mental illness itself and what is the side effect of the medication that the new or expectant mother is taking for the mental illness. There are obviously also clear ethical concerns with being able to design and conduct gold standard or empirical trials into the use of medicines in pregnant women.

Although the lack of research does make it difficult to make specific recommendations, it is generally suggested that haloperidol and olanzapine may be the safest of the antipsychotics for use in pregnant women as they are less likely to cause defects in the unborn baby. However, the mother's health must be assessed as well as the risks to her unborn baby; as discussed above, these medicines can have severe cardiotoxic effects. Robakis and Williams (2013) also suggest that quetiapine may be a good choice if a new or expectant mother requires antipsychotic drug treatment, although the evidence base is scarce. It should be noted that there is a significant association between the atypical antipsychotic medicines and gestational diabetes. There is not such an association between typical antipsychotic medicines and gestational diabetes, which may be an additional consideration when looking at the treatment for expectant mothers at risk of developing this. All pregnant women who take atypical antipsychotics should have regular blood glucose monitoring in addition to their other health checks for this reason.

In relation to breastfeeding, there are risks that any psychiatric medication can be passed through the breast milk from mother to baby, and so any new mother who is planning to breastfeed should talk to a specialist doctor to find out the specific risks of their medication in relation to breast milk. In general, manufacturers of the atypical antipsychotics warn that women should not breastfeed when they are taking these medications. It is less clear for the typical antipsychotics. Any conversations around breastfeeding need to be handled sensitively because deciding on whether or not to breastfeed may be a large and emotional step for the new mother.

CONSIDERATIONS FOR DIFFERENT AGE GROUPS

Older adults

Antipsychotic medication is sometimes used as part of a specialist treatment plan for dementia, especially for those who have delusions or hallucinations as part of their presentation, but this can come with significant complexities and risks (see Chapter 7).

Of course, there are also older adults (people over 65) who may have lived with a psychotic illness for many years and may have an existing treatment plan in place which includes the use of antipsychotics for this purpose. Some older adults may also experience psychotic symptoms as part of a severe depression, and antipsychotics can also be used as a treatment plan in this situation. Alexopoulos et al. (2004) suggests that first-line options for this age group could be risperidone, quetiapine and olanzapine, and aripiprazole as a second line.

With all older adults, any sudden onset of, or change to known psychotic-type symptoms needs a full physical health investigation, and the person's level of cognitive functioning also needs to be considered.

When giving any medication to an older adult, the risk of physical health complications needs to be considered, especially for those with long-term health conditions and/or frailty, and medicines that may cause drowsiness, disorientation and confusion should be avoided as they can increase risk of falls.

Children and young people

In 2013, NICE issued a 'do not do' recommendation, which states that antipsychotic medication in children and young people with a first presentation of sustained psychotic symptoms should not be started in primary care unless it is done in consultation with a consultant psychiatrist with training in child and adolescent mental health.

NICE guideline CG155 covers the use of antipsychotic medication in children and young people, and this was last updated in 2016. These guidelines state that antipsychotic medication must not be used in cases of possible psychosis, and psychological interventions and family interventions should be offered. In confirmed first episode psychosis cases, following a full history, mental health assessment, physical health assessment and discussion with the person and their family, medication may be used. These should usually be the atypical (newer) medications, and the particular risk of increased weight gain with olanzapine must be considered before this drug is chosen. For subsequent episodes, medication can be used and the treatment options should be based on possible risks, physical health history and the history of what worked well previously. NICE (2016) also notes that for those in the 15–17 age bracket who have early indications of schizophrenia, aripiprazole may be used in those intolerant to or unable to take risperidone.

The importance of ongoing family work and access to psychological interventions is also noted, as is the use of creative therapies using the arts.

For children and young people who do not respond to treatment, if the sequential use of adequate doses of at least two different antipsychotic drugs, each used for six to eight weeks, is not effective, then treatment with clozapine may be considered. If this is still not effective, a second antipsychotic (that does not worsen the clozapine side effects) may be used to augment treatment, trialled for up to eight to ten weeks with continuous review and support.

LEARNING FROM A CASE STUDY: TEST YOUR KNOWLEDGE

Tom is a 29-year-old man who is taking 200mg clozapine daily. He takes 75mg in the morning and 125mg at night. Tom has been on this medication for about two years, and it has worked really well for him. He previously took olanzapine 20mg and haloperidol 7mg, but neither of these worked for him. Tom has just returned from a holiday in Turkey with his boyfriend and asks to meet with you as the community psychiatric nurse (CPN) from his community mental health team (CMHT) as he needs an urgent prescription. Tom would like to know if there is a clozapine depot available that he can have instead because he says that it was embarrassing

(Continued)

taking tablets on holiday. He tells you that when he was on holiday, he lost a few tablets as they fell out of the packet, so he has not had a dose for three days, but he is happy to pick up his prescription and take a tablet again today. Tom also tells you that he has not opened his bowels for seven days and he thinks that this is due to the 'funny food' abroad, in addition to the fact that he bought several boxes of cigarettes from duty free and was smoking 'twice as much as normal' whilst on holiday.

1   Is there a depot alternative to clozapine available for Tom?
2   What might be your concerns around Tom missing three days' worth of medication? What needs to happen?
3   Are there any concerns in relation to Tom's sudden increased smoking level?
4   Do you have any other concerns about Tom's health at the moment?

IF I REMEMBER 5 THINGS FROM THIS CHAPTER ...

1   There are two different families of antipsychotic medication, 'typical' and 'atypical'. The typical medications refer to the older medicines and the atypical medications refer to the newer medicines.
2   Some antipsychotic medications are available as long-acting injections. These are called 'depot medications'.
3   Clozapine is an antipsychotic medication that can be used if people do not respond to a minimum of two other antipsychotic medications (at least one to be atypical). It is associated with some serious side effects, and so has its own set of monitoring procedures.
4   Typical antipsychotic medications are strongly linked to EPSE side effects, whereas atypical antipsychotics are more likely to be linked with metabolic side effects.
5   All antipsychotic medications are linked to blood disorders. NMS is the most severe of these and can be fatal if not identified early.

ANSWERS TO THE CASE STUDY QUESTIONS

1   There is no depot alternative to clozapine at the moment. You could discuss trying a different medication in depot form with Tom, but this is unlikely to be effective for him as he has not responded well to both typical and atypical oral treatments other than clozapine.

2   As Tom has missed more than two days of clozapine treatment, he must not start taking his usual dose again. He needs to be retitrated on his clozapine. You need to speak to the team doctor to get this titration arranged immediately. Tom will need close monitoring and weekly blood tests during this time.

3   Yes. A sudden increase in Tom's smoking may have led to changes in how much clozapine was in his blood. You need to talk to Tom about how much he plans to smoke now that he is back in the UK and explain that he should not suddenly increase or decrease his smoking level without discussing it with a healthcare professional.

4   Yes. One concern is the fact that Tom has not opened his bowels for seven days. This indicates constipation. This may be linked to his clozapine, as well as his change in diet whilst on holiday. You need to speak with the team doctor about starting Tom on laxative medication and also arrange for an examination. You should also ask Tom to keep a stool chart so that you can be aware of his bowel habits and constipation and review this with him in a few days' time, as well as giving him advice to help with his constipation, such as encouraging him to increase his fibre intake and level of exercise to stimulate the bowel. It would also be helpful to have a general chat with Tom about how his holiday went and if he has any health concerns, be these sunburn, sexual health or other matters.

REFERENCES AND RECOMMENDED READING

Alexopoulos, G., Streim, J., Carpenter, D., et al. (2004) 'Using antipsychotic agents in older patients', *Journal of Clinical Psychiatry*, 65 (supplement 2): 5–99.

Allison, D.B., Newcomer, J.W., Dunn, A.L., et al. (2009) 'Obesity among those with mental disorders: A National Institute of Mental Health meeting report', *American Journal of Preventative Medicine*, 36 (4): 341–50.

Babu, G.N., Desai, G. and Chandra, P.S. (2015) 'Antipsychotics in pregnancy and lactation', *Indian Journal of Psychiatry*, 57: 303–7.

Collins, E., Drake, M. and Deacon, M. (2013) *The Physical Care of People with Mental Health Problems: A Guide for Best Practice.* London: Sage.

Dixon, M. and Dada, C. (2014) 'How clozapine patients can be monitored safely and effectively', *Clinical Pharmacist.* Available at: https://pharmaceutical-journal.com/article/ld/how-clozapine-patients-can-be-monitored-safely-and-effectively (accessed 1 October 2021).

Glassman, A.H. and Bigger, J.T., Jr (2001) 'Antipsychotic drugs: Prolonged QTc interval, torsade de pointes, and sudden death', *American Journal of Psychiatry*, 158 (11): 1774–82.

Green, L., Vais, A and Harding, K. (2013) 'Preconception care for women with mental health conditions', *British Journal of Hospital Medicines*, 74 (6): 319–22.

Jethwa, K.D. (2018) 'Pharmacological management of antipsychotic-induced akathisia: An update and treatment algorithm', *BJPsych Advances*, 21 (5): 342–4. Available at: www.cambridge.org/core/journals/bjpsych-advances/article/pharmacological-management-of-antipsychoticinduced-akathisia-an-update-and-treatment-algorithm/F9539508CAF512358754C6FD93BAF26D (accessed 2 July 2021).

Mind (2020) 'Antipsychotics'. Available at: www.mind.org.uk/information-support/drugs-and-treatments/antipsychotics/about-antipsychotics/?o=7290#.WA97SE0UWmM (accessed 1 October 2021).

Moncrieff, J. (2008) *The Myth of the Chemical Cure*. Basingstoke: Palgrave Macmillan.

NICE (2013) 'Do not do recommendation'. Available at: www.nice.org.uk/donotdo/antipsychotic-medication-in-children-and-young-people-with-a-first-presentation-ofsustained-psychotic-symptoms-should-not-be-started-in-primary-care-unless-it-is-donein-consultation-with-a-consultant (accessed 2 July 2021).

NICE (2016) 'Psychosis and schizophrenia in children and young people: recognition and management'. Available at: www.nice.org.uk/guidance/cg155/chapter/Recommendations#possible-psychosis (accessed 2 July 2021).

NMC (2015, updated 2018) *The Code*. Available at: www.nmc.org.uk/globalassets/sitedocuments/nmc-publications/nmc-code.pdf (accessed 1 October 2021).

Pies, R.W. (2011) 'Psychiatry's new brain–mind and the legend of the "chemical imbalance"', *Psychiatric Times*. Available at: www.psychiatrictimes.com/view/psychiatrys-new-brain-mind-and-legend-chemical-imbalance (accessed 1 October 2021).

Robakis, T. and Williams, K. (2013) 'Atypical antipsychotics during pregnancy', *Current Psychiatry*, 12 (7): 12–18.

Tschoner, A., Engl, J., Laimer, M., et al. (2007) 'Metabolic side effects of antipsychotic medication', *International Journal of Clinical Practice*, 61 (8): 1356–70.

Waddell, L. and Taylor, M. (2008) 'A new self-rating scale for detecting atypical or second-generation antipsychotic side effects', *Journal of Psychopharmacology*, 22 (3): 238–33.

6 MEDICINES FOR RAPID TRANQUILLISATION

LIZ HOLLAND

AFTER READING THIS CHAPTER, YOU WILL BE ABLE TO:

- Know what the term 'rapid tranquillisation' means, and be aware of the different stages of rapid tranquillisation
- Understand what we mean by the concept of 'PRN' medication
- Consider the risks associated with rapid tranquillisation interventions
- Undertake clinical decision-making around rapid tranquillisation situations
- Demonstrate an awareness of the different types of medicines available for rapid tranquillisation

---

WHAT DO WE MEAN BY 'RAPID TRANQUILLISATION'?

NICE (2015) defines 'rapid tranquillisation' as a situation in which medicine is given to a person who is very agitated or displaying aggressive behaviour in order to help calm them down quickly. This is to reduce any risk to themselves or others, and to enable them to receive the care that they need. It is important when you commence in a new organisation that you look at their policy around rapid tranquillisation so you understand precisely what constitutes rapid tranquillisation within the organisation, and how it is differentiated from PRN medication.

'Rapid tranquillisation' is a serious and high-risk intervention as it involves giving powerful medication to sedate a vulnerable person, and these medications can have severe side effects. Additionally, rapid tranquillisation medicines are often given in psychiatric emergency situations, and in these situations patients may not consent to medicinal intervention, which means that physical restraint interventions may need to be used in order to ensure the safety of the patient, the safety of the people around them and to enable the rapid tranquillisation medication to be given. The potential risks around restraint will be discussed later in the chapter. Due to the level of risk involved, rapid tranquillisation should only be given as a last resort, when all verbal interventions to help to calm the patient have failed, or in high risk, unprecedented emergency situations when immediate intervention is required to maintain safety. Rapid tranquillisation and restraint interventions are used across mental health services, police custody services and prison services.

- If you are working in a mental health setting in which rapid tranquillisation may be given, it is important to have a basic understanding of mental health law and legislation. All mental health law and legislation is linked to the Human Rights Act, and the ways in which we give rapid tranquillisation and use restraint can seem to be impacting on the human rights of individuals, particularly around their liberty, freedom and choice. The Human Rights Act is what we call a 'foundation law', which means that the way in which any other law is written or applied must comply with it. Any use of the Mental Health Act 1983 (MHA) must be treated in this way as it legislates clear ways in which a person's liberty may be restricted and how this must be done safely. In practice this means:
- A person cannot be 'detained' without good reason, and that this reason must be linked to harm to the person or those around them.
- If a person is detained under the MHA, the person's human rights means that the legislation of the MHA must be followed in order to ensure clear justification and fair and legal treatment.
- The person has the right to be given information on why they have been detained (in a way that they can understand), to understand their rights, and understand how they can challenge the reasons for their detention.

When we apply this to decision-making to go ahead with a rapid tranquillisation intervention, we should consider the questions below to ensure that we are practising in a way that is informed by human rights:

- Is it lawful? For example, is giving someone treatment against their will justified by legislation such as the MHA or the Mental Capacity Act 2005 (MCA)? Or is there a significant and immediate risk to life?
- Is there a legitimate reason? For example, are you making the decision because you are trying to prevent harm?

- Is it proportionate? For example, have you tried talking to the person and all other less restrictive options, and is this the most proportionate action given the level of risk? Have you talked with any family or friend carers to help you understand the situation?

GO FURTHER ...

If you would like to read more around mental health law and legislation, it is recommended that you read the book by Murphy and Wales (2013), *Mental Health Law in Nursing*. Please note that the examples in this chapter use the Mental Health Act references which cover England and Wales. If you are in a different part of the UK (or working with individuals who may be from a different part of the UK and may be used to being treated under a different part of the Act), you may want to familiarize yourself with:

- The Mental Health (Care and Treatment) (Scotland) Act 2003
- The Mental Health Act Ireland (2001)
- The Mental Health Act (Nothern Ireland) Order (1986)

If you are interested in learning more about human rights and how they apply to the care, treatment and decisions made in mental healthcare, see the British Institute of Human Rights website www.bihr.org.uk/resources-for-service-providers, which is brilliant.

Another useful document is the Mental Unites (Use of Force) Act 2018. This provides the statutory guidance NHS organisations in England and police forces in England and Wales must follow when using force. This comes from significant engagement with different groups and perspectives of people, learning from tragedy and trauma and a desire to improve the experience of care to those who may be at risk of needing physical interventions to maintain safety when receiving care. This is available via: https://www.gov.uk/government/publications/mental-health-units-use-of-force-act-2018/mental-health-units-use-of-force-act-2018-statutory-guidance-for-nhs-organisations-in-england-and-police-forces-in-england-and-wales

---

A general rule is that rapid tranquillisation and restraint interventions should not be used on informal patients. This is because these patients have the capacity and the right to make decisions around their treatment, and so treatment should not be forced on them. The violation of their human right to liberty is not covered by another law. The only exception to this rule may be if there is a sudden and immediate risk to human life, in which case any necessary (and proportionate) intervention can be justified under common law. If an informal patient is subject to rapid tranquillisation or restraint, or is likely to need these interventions, it may be necessary to assess for an 'emergency section' under the MHA. If a patient is already detained under the MHA, then they may be subject to rapid tranquillisation and restraint interventions even without their consent, but only if the intervention is in the best interests of the patient and is preventing a significant risk of harm to them or to others.

THE FIVE STAGES OF RAPID TRANQUILLISATION

Every organisation will have its own policy around the use of rapid tranquillisation and restraint interventions and, although this will be based largely on the NICE guidelines for the management of violence and aggression (2015), there may be local differences which you need to be aware of, and so it is strongly recommended that you read your organisation's policy in conjunction with this chapter. However, it is generally recognised that there are five stages in rapid tranquillisation interventions.

Stage one: Verbal de-escalation

This first stage of working with anyone who is highly distressed is the most important as it is the least restrictive. Verbal de-escalation should always be attempted before medication is used. This stage involves simply talking with the person who is highly distressed. You should be thinking about:

- What is it that might be upsetting the patient? Can you identify any triggers?
- Is the patient able to explain what is going on? Can you make sense of the situation?
- Can you distract the patient from the situation that is causing upset?
- Are you able to use negotiation or find a solution to the problem?
- Empathise! Can you 'agree to disagree' on something?
- Is the patient willing to move with you to a quieter area?
- Would the patient be better cared for in a lower-stimulus environment, such as a psychiatric intensive care unit (PICU)?
- Could enhanced observations be used to support the patient?

Stage two: Use of oral medication

If you have worked through all of the above and the patient's level of distress is not improving, you now need to think about whether some 'calm down' medication may be beneficial to help reduce the patient's agitation. This may be a benzodiazepine (e.g. lorazepam), sedating antihistamine (e.g. promethazine) or an antipsychotic (e.g. haloperidol). The medicines list below discusses these options in more depth. When deciding what medicine to give, how you have this conversation with the patient is really important. You will need to explain exactly what the medicine is you would like them to take, what the dose is, why you would like them to take it and how it might make them feel. For example:

> Joe, I am really worried that you are becoming very upset. I saw you kicking the chair in the dining room and I saw you swearing at Amar. I am worried that if we don't help you to become less upset, you might end up hurting yourself or hurting Amar and I do not want that to happen. These two blue tablets are called 'promethazine', and there is 50mg here, which is a typical dose. It is a medicine that can help you feel calm and less upset very quickly. It can sometimes also make you feel a bit sleepy after you take it, but a nurse will stay with you to make sure that you are OK. Do you have any questions?

Medication taken orally takes around 30 minutes to demonstrate an effect but the fullness of the stomach can have an effect: the fuller the stomach, the slower the rate of absorption.

Stage three: Use of injectable (intramuscular) medication

If the patient has accepted the oral medication at stage two, you should wait 45 minutes (if it is safe to do so) to assess their initial response to the oral medication. If oral medication has not had the desired effect after 45 minutes but the patient remains agreeable, try a second oral medication. If this second oral medication is not effective, you may need to move to an injectable. You may also need to move straight to an injectable rapid tranquillisation medication if the patient is refusing to take any oral medication, or in extreme cases of distress where there is an imminent risk of harm. If the patient is refusing medication you may need to use a physical restraint intervention in order to hold the patient and safely administer the injection. The rapid tranquillisation medicines that can be given as IM injections are largely the same as those that are given orally. It is usually considered best practice to use an injection of a benzodiazepine or sedating antihistamine before moving to an IM antipsychotic, due to the risks of side effects. Lorazepam and promethazine are often the most commonly used first-line injectable medicines. Usually, one IM medication is given, and response is assessed after 30 minutes before a decision is made about whether further medication is needed. In extreme distress and agitation, two IM injections can be given at once, each containing a different medication, but this should be assessed and prescribed explicitly by a doctor. Always remember to reassure the patient and explain exactly what has been happening. Medication administered by IM injection typically takes 15–30 minutes to have an effect and this time is affected by factors such as the patient's weight and level of movement.

Stage four: Repeat injectable (intramuscular) medication

If you are in a psychiatric emergency situation where you are considering giving a second rapid tranquillisation injection, you should have a doctor present. You must also ensure that you have staff trained in both medical and psychiatric emergency interventions. You must wait at least 30 minutes between giving the first injection and the second injection, and these injections should be different medications where possible (unless there is a partial response to the first injection – more details later in the chapter). For example, if you give lorazepam 2mg as the first injection and the patient remains highly distressed after 30 minutes, you may then choose to give promethazine 50mg as the second injection. Antipsychotic IM medications are often used as the second-line choice for rapid tranquillisation, depending on the patient's cardiac status.

Stage five: Long-acting sedatives

In very serious and severe cases of acute agitation, a long-acting sedative may be considered. These are always given as IM injections. A senior pharmacist and a consultant psychiatrist should always be involved in any decisions around the use of a long-acting sedative. These should never be used on a long-term basis. Zuclopenthixol acetate (Acuphase) is the most well known of the long-acting sedatives. This has an initial strong sedative effect shortly, but not immediately (two to eight hours), after it is first administered, and a residual sedative and antipsychotic effect that lasts for two to three days following administration. This should never be given to a patient who has not previously been exposed to antipsychotic medication.

HOW DO I DECIDE WHAT MEDICINE TO CHOOSE TO GIVE FOR RAPID TRANQUILLISATION?

Working in psychiatric emergency situations can be highly stressful and it is really important to seek support and supervision following your involvement in these situations. Many of the decisions around rapid tranquillisation medicines and emergency interventions are nurse-led; it is usual practice that psychiatric doctors will prescribe different medicines that can be used for rapid tranquillisation on a patient's drug chart, and in this situation, the nurse will look at the options available and choose the most appropriate one. The nurse may also be in a situation where they need to decide on what dose should be given. Previous experience and sharing ideas with your colleagues will always be helpful here, but current research shows that there is no evidence that higher doses of rapid tranquillisation medications cause more rapid or effective sedation (Calver et al., 2013), and you should therefore always go for the lower dose if you are unsure.

When working in emergency situations, it is also very helpful to think about the potential use of illicit drugs and alcohol; you need to consider if they could be contributing to the sudden change in the patient's behaviour. If you think that the patient has or may have consumed drugs or alcohol, find out what has been consumed (if possible) and then seek advice from a doctor or pharmacist before giving any medication; there may be contraindications between the alcohol and drugs that the patient has used and those that you are about to give. For example, benzodiazepines such as lorazepam can slow a person's respiration rate and so you would not want to give them to someone who drank a large amount of alcohol, as this also slows down a person's breathing.

A simple rule to remember with rapid tranquillisation is that if you have not seen a recent ECG for the patient, you should never give them any sort of antipsychotic medication as rapid tranquillisation. This is because antipsychotic medications, particularly when used in emergency situations, can affect the rhythm of the heart, and this can cause serious complications and even death. Additionally, antipsychotic medications should only be used for rapid tranquillisation in patients who have previously been exposed to antipsychotic drug treatment.

It is also important to take into account a patient's regular medication and the medication prescribed for 'as required', which is where the prescription for any rapid tranquillisation medication will appear on a drug chart. For example, if a patient is prescribed 25mg promethazine three times a day on a regular basis (75mg total) and the 24-hour maximum written is 100mg, then you cannot give an extra 50mg promethazine for rapid tranquillisation. It would therefore be best to select an alternative medicine such as lorazepam.

Rund et al. (2006) support the use of lorazepam as the first-choice drug for rapid tranquillisation, saying that the associated risks are usually minimal when it is used for single-dose or short-term administration.

It is suggested that you look at your local policy on rapid tranquillisation and speak to your consultant and your pharmacist in order to see what the preferred rapid tranquillisation medicines are in your area of work. However, the NICE guidelines on the management of violence and aggression (2015) do make some suggestions, although these are not mandatory and may need to be adapted due to individual patient needs. These guidelines suggest that you use lorazepam as your first-line response for rapid tranquillisation as this is the safest option. For a second-line intervention, they suggest giving a combination of haloperidol and promethazine together if the patient has a current ECG available that shows a normal heart rhythm. If an ECG is not available or is indicative of any cardiac problems, you may need to consider a second dose of lorazepam if there has been a partial response to the first dose, or promethazine alone if there was no response to the initial lorazepam.

PRONE RESTRAINT

It was horrific ... I had some bad experiences of being restrained face down with my face pushed into a pillow ... I can't begin to describe how scary it was, not being able to signal, communicate, breathe or speak ... Anything you do to try to communicate, they put more pressure on you. The more you try to signal, the worse it is. (Service user quote from the Mind report on prone restraint, 2013)

As you can see from the above quote, having to go through a restraint intervention can be an incredibly traumatic and emotive experience for the patient, even if it is the best interest intervention at the time. It is therefore very important to debrief the patient after the restraint has taken place and the person has become less distressed.

The prone position refers to a restraint position in which the patient is held with their torso and head pointing towards the floor. The prone restraint system is a very high-risk restraint position due to the fact that the person being restrained may have pressure applied to their chest, and compression to the chest may cause problems with the airway and/or the cardiac system (Department of Health, 2014). It is important that alternatives to prone restraint are considered wherever possible. Sadly, Mind (2013) found that deaths caused by the prone position are not uncommon. In 2011, in the UK, eight people detained under the Mental Health Act 1983 died in the prone position. In 2013, there were three such individuals who died and a further thousand were physically injured in restraint incidents, and this is only from available and recorded data. Haddad and Anderson (2002) additionally note that when prone restraint is used in conjunction with an IM injectable antipsychotic, the risk of the person developing a fatal arrhythmia increases. This is why the government is aiming to support all mental health and learning disability services to eliminate prone restraint. Front-line staff are being trained in the use of 'safer alternative restraint positions'. The use of supine restraint (person on their back) is being used more frequently, and it is possible to administer medication in this position by pulling the leg across the body to allow access to the dorsogluteal muscle. To date there is not a large body of evidence around the risks associated with supine restraint.

POSSIBLE COMPLICATIONS THAT CAN ARISE FOLLOWING RAPID TRANQUILLISATION

There are many complications that can arise in patients who have taken medication for the purposes of rapid tranquillisation, which is why post-intervention care, observation and monitoring are so important (see below). Overall, the most common concern is to do with respiration; because the medications we give people for rapid tranquillisation are designed to make them feel calm and sleepy, they can reduce an individual's respiration rate. If someone is taking in fewer breaths or their breaths are less deep, then they will take in less oxygen, which may consequently affect their oxygen saturations. Research by Calver et al. (2013) suggests that low oxygen levels (oxygen desaturation) and low blood pressure (hypotension) are the most commonly seen adverse effects following rapid tranquillisation, and these become more severe when higher doses of medication are given. When antipsychotic medication is used for rapid tranquillisation, there are particular concerns around cardiac complications as these drugs can affect the electrical rhythm of the heart, especially around something known as the QTc interval. If the electrical rhythm of the heart is disrupted, then the person will suffer an abnormal heart rhythm, the most concerning of which is **ventricular fibrillation**. This can lead to a cardiac arrest situation and possible resulting death. There are individual risk factors that may make a patient more likely to suffer a serious reaction to antipsychotic medication given for rapid tranquillisation. These include:

- If the injection is given under restraint
- A slow metabolism
- Being female
- Being an older adult
- An existing electrolyte imbalance
- Existing cardiac problems
- **Hepatic** or **renal impairments**. (Haddad and Anderson, 2002)

An additional side effect that you may see after administering an injectable antipsychotic is severe muscle stiffness. A medication called procyclidine can be used to alleviate this. In patients who are particularly sensitive to this side effect, procyclidine can be given as an injection alongside the antipsychotic.

Acute dystonia can be another side effect we see when antipsychotic medication is given for rapid tranquillisation, both orally and via IM. Acute dystonia is a movement disorder where the muscles contract involuntarily, and this leads to abnormal postures, expressions and movements; with anti-psychotic medications the most common issues can be with the eyes and the mouth and tongue. This response tends to come within three to four days of the medication being given, and is most common in younger people (under 45) and men (Loonen and Ivanova, 2020). It is something that can be very distressing to see and causes significant panic and worry to the person experiencing it, as they can feel out of control. If this happens, give the person lots of reassurance and ensure they are not receiving any further medication of the same type. Procyclidine is usually an effective treatment and should be given as soon as possible. The risk of acute dystonia is particularly prevalent with haloperidol and so procyclidine IM should usually be prescribed at the same time as the haloperidol IM, and discuss as a team if you may want to give both of these at the same time to reduce the risk. There can be other emergency treatment options depending on the person's reaction, and so a consultant review is important in these situations.

It is therefore very important to complete full physical monitoring of your patients as soon as you are able to, so that you have information regarding the risk factors listed above.

NURSING CARE POST-RAPID TRANQUILLISATION

As rapid tranquillisation is classed as a 'high-risk intervention', there are several care requirements that nurses must follow after the intervention has finished:

- Any patient who has received rapid tranquillisation (oral or injection) should have a full set of vital signs (blood pressure, pulse, oxygen satura-tions, respiration rate, temperature and level of consciousness assessment using the 'alert, voice, pain, unresponsive' or AVPU scale) recorded imme-diately following the intervention. These observations should typically be taken every 15 minutes for the first hour following rapid tranquillisation if the patient is agreeable. If the patient does not agree, then it is important to document that the physical observations were offered but refused, and then to keep trying! If the patient declines all physical monitoring, the minimum you can do is to note an observation of the patient's physical state from what you are able to see from a distance, such as whether the patient's skin has an altered appearance, what their breathing is like, how alert they are, how they are behaving at the moment. These are known as non-contact observations. An ECG may be required following rapid tranquillisation for some patients, especially those taking regular antipsychotic medication and/or those with existing cardiac concerns. Physical monitoring should then continue on an hourly basis until a senior nurse or a doctor makes the decision that there are no further concerns about the patient's physical health at this time. Every organisation will have a clear protocol for post-rapid-tranquillisation monitoring, so it is important that you are aware of this.

- The patient's care plan and risk assessment should always be updated after rapid tranquillisation. If possible, it is always best to do these together with the patient after you have completed the debrief with them. The NICE guidelines on violence and aggression (2015) suggest a framework for this debrief if you would like support on how to structure it.
- A senior medical review should always be arranged within 72 hours of an incident in which a patient required rapid tranquillisation. The NICE guidelines on violence and aggression (2015) also recommend that any patient receiving rapid tranquillisation should have a daily review of their medicines.
- Ensure that both the patient and the staff team involved in the intervention receive a full debrief following the incident. Any visitors or other people on the ward who saw the incident should also be offered a debrief. The person's family or friend carers must also be informed if they are involved in the person's care.
- Documentation of the rapid tranquillisation event and intervention is really important. The incident should be recorded both as an incident report using your local system, and as an entry in the patient notes. These records must include exactly what happened, what medication was given and at what time and what dose, which staff were involved and what role they played in the intervention, how the patient was before, during and after the incident, what physical observations have been taken and what the readings are, and any residual concerns regarding the patient.
- Fluid monitoring should be considered for the patient, if appropriate.

THE MEDICINES LIST

This medicines list will cover the most commonly used medications in rapid tranquillisation. It is not an exhaustive list and it is really important that you look at your local policy and recommendations, as first-line recommendations may differ slightly in different services and organisations. It is also important that you keep up to date with recommendations and research in this area, as guidelines frequently change.

This medicines list discusses rapid tranquillisation medications that can be given in both oral and injectable form, and divides medicines into four classifications: antihistamine medications, benzodiazepines, antipsychotic medications and long-acting sedatives.

Antihistamine medications

Antihistamine medications work by interacting with histamine receptors found in the immune system, which can reduce inflammation. In mental health treatments, they are often used as sedatives because they can cause extreme drowsiness when taken.

The key side effects for sedative antihistamines are drowsiness, headaches, a dry mouth, gastrointestinal upsets, blurred vision and **urinary retention**.

Drug name: **Promethazine**

UK brand names: Sominex, Phenergan

Average doses:

- Oral: 25–50mg
- Emergency injection: 25–50mg
- Total maximum dose by both forms within 24 hours: 100mg

What form does it come in? Tablet, liquid, solution for emergency injection

Does it interact with any other medications: Yes. The following interactions are known:

- *Tricyclic antidepressants*: There is an increased risk of antimuscarinic side effects if these are taken with promethazine
- *MAOI*: Promethazine should never be taken alongside an MAOI

Additional information:

- Promethazine is available over the counter without a prescription
- Promethazine is also licensed for use as a sleep aid, for use in allergies such as hayfever and for emergency treatment of anaphylaxis, although doses are different in these areas.

Benzodiazepine medications

Benzodiazepine medications work on a brain transmitter called gamma-aminobutyric acid (GABA). The role of GABA is to reduce the brain's ability to develop memories, produce emotion, engage in rational thought and promote breathing. Benzodiazepines work by increasing GABA levels in the brain, and these functions are therefore reduced when someone takes benzodiazepines. Consequently, they can cause extreme drowsiness, which is why they are used for sedation. However, the fact that benzodiazepines can slow down breathing is quite concerning, and so any patient who is given a benzodiazepine should have their respiration rate monitored in order to ensure that it remains within normal limits. You should not give benzodiazepines to any patient whom you suspect has consumed alcohol, as this also slows down breathing.

Benzodiazepines are highly addictive. This is because, over time, the brain can become used to their effects. It means that increasingly higher doses are needed in order to achieve the same effects. Benzodiazepines should therefore be prescribed only for very short periods of time.

The key side effects of benzodiazepines, alongside the severe risk of respiratory depression, are drowsiness, dizziness, headaches, problems getting an erection, feeling wobbly on your feet, feeling generally unwell and a feeling of weakness in your muscles.

(Continued)

Drug name: Lorazepam

UK brand names: Ativan

Average doses:

- Oral: 1–2mg
- Emergency injection: 1–2mg
- Total maximum dose by both forms within 24 hours: 4mg

What form does it come in? Tablet, solution for emergency injection

Does it interact with any other medications: Yes. The following interactions are known:

- *All antipsychotic medication*: Taking any antipsychotic alongside lorazepam can increase sedation
- *Mirtazapine*: Taking mirtazapine alongside lorazepam can increase sedation
- *Tricyclic antidepressants*: Taking any tricyclic antidepressants alongside lorazepam can increase sedative effects
- *Valproate*: Valproate is known to increase the blood level of lorazepam
- *Clozapine*: There is a significant concern that if someone on clozapine takes lorazepam, respiratory arrest is more likely, a drop in blood pressure is likely and cardiac arrest is more likely.

Additional information:

- Caffeine should be avoided as this can decrease the efficacy of lorazepam
- Grapefruit juice should be avoided as this can increase the efficacy of lorazepam

Drug name: Clonazepam

UK brand names: None

Average doses:

- Oral: 2–5mg
- Total maximum within 24 hours: 10mg

What form does it come in? Tablet and liquid

Does it interact with any other medications: Yes. The following interactions are known:

- *All antipsychotic medication*: Taking any antipsychotic alongside clonazepam can increase sedation
- *Valproate*: Valproate can decrease the blood level of clonazepam
- *Carbamazepine*: Carbamazepine can decrease the blood level of clonazepam
- *Lithium*: If clonazepam is taken alongside lithium, there is an increased risk of severe side effects

Drug name: **Diazepam**

UK brand names: Dialar, Diazemuls, Diazepam Desitin, Diazepam Rectubes, Rimapam, Stesolid, Tensium

Average doses:

- Oral: 5-15mg
- Total maximum within 24 hours: 30mg

What form does it come in? Tablet, liquid, solution for injection and rectal tubes. However, in rapid tranquillisation, only the oral forms (tablet and liquid) are used

Does it interact with any other medications: Yes. The following interactions are known:

- *All antipsychotic medication*: Taking any antipsychotic in addition to diazepam can increase sedation
- *Mirtazapine*: Taking mirtazapine alongside diazepam can increase sedation
- *Tricyclic antidepressants*: Taking any tricyclic antidepressants in con-juction with diazepam can increase sedative effects
- *Fluvoxamine*: Fluvoxamine can increase the blood level of diazepam
- *Zotepine*: Zotepine can increase the blood level of diazepam
- *Valproate*: Valproate can increase the blood level of diazepam

(Continued)

- *Clozapine*: There is a significant concern that if someone on clozapine takes diazepam, respiratory arrest is more likely, a drop in blood pressure is likely and cardiac arrest is more likely
- *Olanzapine*: Giving olanzapine and diazepam together creates a risk of slow respiratory rate, slow heartbeat and low blood pressure

Additional information: Can also be used for alcohol withdrawal

Antipsychotic medications

Remember, antipsychotic medications should only be used for rapid tranquillisation if you know that the person's agitation or distress is being caused by a psychotic illness, and you have a current ECG for the person that shows that they do not have any cardiac concerns. The person must also have previously tolerated some form of antipsychotic medication without a severe reaction.

To read more about antipsychotic medications, see Chapter 5, where the side effects for antipsychotic medications and the different types of antipsychotics are covered in detail.

Drug name: Haloperidol

UK brand names: Dozic, Haldol, Serenace

Average doses:

- Oral: 1-3mg up to three times daily
- Emergency injection: 0.75-5mg up to three times daily
- Total daily recommended maximum: 20mg if taken orally and 12mg if taken by injection

What form does it come in? Tablet, liquid, solution for emergency injection

Does it interact with any other medications: Yes. The following interactions are known:

- *Carbamazepine*: Carbamazepine can reduce blood level of haloperidol

- *Chlorpromazine*: If chlorpromazine and haloperidol are taken together, the blood levels of haloperidol may increase
- *Clozapine*: Clozapine and haloperidol depot should not be given together as there is a risk of blood disorder, and treatment cannot be stopped quickly should this occur
- *Fluoxetine*: If fluoxetine and haloperidol are taken together, the blood levels of haloperidol may increase
- *Fluvoxamine*: If fluvoxamine and haloperidol are taken together, the blood levels of haloperidol may increase
- *Lithium*: Taking lithium and haloperidol together increases the risk of NMS
- *SSRI antidepressants*: If taken with haloperidol, these can lead to an increased risk of serious disturbances of heart rhythm
- *Sulpiride*: If taken with haloperidol, there is an increased risk of irregular heartbeat
- *Tricyclic antidepressants*: If taken with haloperidol, these can lead to an increased risk of serious disturbances of heart rhythm
- *Venlafaxine*: If venlafaxine and haloperidol are taken together, the blood levels of haloperidol may increase

Additional information:

- Also available to be given as a depot
- Typical antipsychotic

Drug name: Olanzapine

UK brand names: Zalasta, Zyprexa

Average doses:

- Oral: 5-10mg daily
- Emergency injection: 10mg, which can be repeated once if required
- Total daily recommended maximum in all forms: 20mg

What form does it come in? Tablet, orodispersible tablet, solution for emergency injection

(Continued)

Does it interact with any other medications: Yes. The following interactions are known:

- *Benzodiazepines given by IM*: If given together, there is an increased risk of low blood pressure, low pulse and low respiration rate
- *Carbamazepine*: Carbamazepine can reduce the blood level of olanzapine
- *Fluvoxamine*: Fluvoxamine can increase plasma levels of olanzapine
- *Lithium*: Taking olanzapine alongside lithium increases the risk of lithium toxicity
- *Valproate*: Taking valproate with olanzapine can increase the risk of a reduced white blood cell count

Additional information:

- Also available to be given as a depot
- Atypical antipsychotic
- Metabolism of olanzapine is affected by how much the person smokes

Drug name: Risperidone

UK brand names: Risperdal

Average doses:

- Oral: 1–6mg
- Total daily maximum: 16mg

What form does it come in? Tablet, soluble tablet and liquid

Does it interact with any other medications? Yes. The following interactions are known:

- *Carbamazepine*: Carbamazepine can reduce the blood level of risperidone
- *Clozapine*: Clozapine and risperidone depot should not be given together as there is a risk of blood disorder, and treatment cannot be stopped quickly should this occur
- *Fluoxetine*: If fluoxetine and risperidone are taken together, the blood levels of risperidone may increase

- *Lithium*: Taking lithium and risperidone together increases the risk of NMS
- *Paroxetine*: Paroxetine is known to increase the adverse effects of risperidone
- *Tricyclic antidepressants*: If taken with risperidone, these can lead to an increased risk of serious disturbances of heart rhythm

Additional information:

- Also available to be given as a depot
- Atypical antipsychotic

Drug name: Aripiprazole

UK brand names: Abilify

Average doses:

- Oral: 10-15mg
- Emergency injection: 9.75mg, up to three times a day
- Total daily maximum in all forms: 30mg

What form does it come in? Tablet, liquid and solution for emergency injection

Does it interact with any other medications: Yes. The following interactions are known:

- *Carbamazepine*: Carbamazepine can decrease the efficacy of aripiprazole
- *Lorazepam*: If lorazepam and aripiprazole are taken together, then there is an increased risk of low blood pressure
- *SSRI and SNRI antidepressants*: There is an increased risk of serotonin syndrome if these are taken alongside aripiprazole
- *St John's wort*: St John's wort can decrease the efficacy of aripiprazole

Additional information:

- Also available to be given as a depot
- Atypical antipsychotic

(Continued)

Long-acting sedatives (antipsychotic)

Drug name: **Zuclopenthixol acetate**

UK brand names: Clopixol, Acuphase

Average doses: Emergency injection: 50–150mg, with a maximum of four injections to be given in any two-week period

What form does it come in? Solution for emergency injection

Does it interact with any other medications: Yes. The following interactions are known:

- *Clozapine*: A long-acting sedative should not be given with clozapine because if the person responds badly and/or has severe side effects to either drug, treatment cannot be stopped quickly
- *Risperidone*: If given with zuclopenthixol acetate, there is an increased risk of heart problems
- *Tricyclic antidepressants*: If any tricyclic antidepressant is given with zuclopenthixol acetate, there is an increased risk of heart problems
- *Lithium*: If someone on lithium is given zuclopenthixol acetate, there is an increased risk of changes in heart rhythm, movement disorders and NMS

Additional information:

- Once given, this medication will remain in the person's system for about 19 days
- The emergency injection solution contains coconut oil, so be aware of allergy status
- Typical antipsychotic

RAPID TRANQUILLISATION IN PREGNANT WOMEN AND BREASTFEEDING MOTHERS

Working with new and expectant mothers in high levels of distress can be a very emotional experience for all those involved, not least the patient and their family. There is very limited research and evidence for the use of rapid tranquillisation in this client group, and so it is hard to draw any clear conclusions about recommendations in this area. It is, however, recommended that when considering a rapid tranquillisation intervention for a new or expectant mother you exhaust all other options first, and then undertake a careful consideration of all the risks and benefits that you are aware of in relation to subjecting the woman to the intervention. You need to be certain that this is the best interest intervention for the woman at this time.

In terms of restraint interventions for this client group, you have to be extremely careful because, if the woman is pregnant, then the restraint intervention could cause harm to the unborn baby, particularly in the third trimester. If the woman is 20 weeks pregnant or more and restraint is required, then she should never be held in the prone position, and the minimum number of people possible should be involved in the restraint so as to reduce unnecessary force. Female staff should be used where possible to preserve dignity. Restraint positions that may be more suitable could be seated restraint, supine restraint (on her back) or on her side. Note that after 16 weeks of pregnancy, women should avoid lying on their back for extended periods, and so a side position is the safest option.

In terms of medication used for rapid tranquillisation for new and expectant mothers, lorazepam is considered the safest choice, within the usual dose ranges. If an injectable antipsychotic is required, haloperidol is the best choice, but a lower dose should be used (2–5mg).

A perinatal psychiatry service should always be involved in treatment plans for new or expectant mothers receiving rapid tranquillisation, and it may also be beneficial to request additional midwifery checks following restraint interventions.

CONSIDERATIONS FOR DIFFERENT AGE GROUPS

Older adults

In older adults, there must be good consideration of the person's physical frailty, any mobility needs and any long-term health matters in any restraint and/or rapid tranquillisation situation. Older adults may need bespoke restraint plans, based on their health and mobility needs.

For adults over 65, the first-line treatment for rapid tranquillisation is lorazepam, but this is at a lower dose than for adults under 65; 0.5mg–1mg, rather than 1mg–2mg. Antipsychotics can also be used if clinically indicated for rapid tranquillisation (see Chapter 5 on antipsychotic medications for specific considerations), with olanzapine being the preferred choice where possible. Doses again may be lower than in adults under 65.

Children and young people

Young people have developing brains, and this means that they are particularly susceptible to side effects from rapid tranquillisation, and so close and careful monitoring post intervention is key, with care and treatment plans being updated after each situation based on what worked well and what did not. A particular side effect to watch out for is the risk of disinhibition after use of benzodiazepines.

Parents and carers should be involved whereever possible, both in planning for situations and in discussing and identifying the learning afterwards.

Lorazepam is generally regarded as the first-line option for rapid tranquillisation in children and young people, and the dose should be prescribed based on the person's age and size. Promethazine may also be able to be used.

The NICE guideline (2016) for treating children and young people with a psychotic illness additionally notes that children and young people may require rapid tranquillisation and restraint when they are highly distressed. The use of antipsychotic medication in these situations requires careful consideration, especially if the person has not previously taken such medication. Young people also have an increased risk of having an acute dystonic reaction (involuntary muscle contractions leading to abnormal movement and posture). Haloperidol in particular should be avoided, and if an IM antipsychotic option is needed, olanzapine may be the first consideration.

LEARNING FROM A CASE STUDY: TEST YOUR KNOWLEDGE

Eric is a 68-year-old man who has a diagnosis of bipolar disorder. He has not had a hospital admission for over 20 years.

Six months ago, Eric suffered a massive heart attack. All of his psychiatric medication was stopped whilst he was in an intensive care unit (ICU). Eric made a full recovery but is still taking cardiac medication. He is obese and suffers from ongoing hypertension.

Eric has recently become manic and hit his wife, which he has never done before. Eric's son panicked as his dad was 'out of control' and called the police. The police arranged a Mental Health Act assessment for Eric as they were concerned that he was 'paranoid and delusional', and he arrived on the acute ward, under section 2 of the MHA 1983, on Saturday afternoon.

Due to his elation, Eric is refusing all physical monitoring, including blood tests and an ECG. He swore at you when you approached him and said that if you do not leave him alone, he will 'knock you out'. He is refusing all treatment and is not sleeping.

You are in ward round on Monday morning and ask the multidisciplinary team (MDT) what to do about Eric. The specialist registrar (SpR), who is chairing the ward round, suggests that you forcibly medicate Eric in order to 'calm him down'. He prescribes lorazepam 2mg (oral and IM) and aripiprazole (an antipsychotic) 9.75mg (oral and IM). He tells you to ensure that Eric gets these medications using 'any method you need to'. Worried, you go to see Eric, and ask him if he will take some tablets from you. At this point, he knocks over a chair, makes a fist and tells you to 'sod off'. Your nursing colleague suggests that you use a rapid tranquillisation intervention at this point:

1   What might be the benefits of giving Eric rapid tranquillisation?
2   What are your concerns around giving Eric rapid tranquillisation?
3   What nursing care would you need to put in place if you decided to give Eric rapid tranquillisation?
4   Would you choose to administer lorazepam or aripiprazole in this situation?

IF I REMEMBER 5 THINGS FROM THIS CHAPTER...

1   Rapid tranquillisation is a last resort intervention used to reduce acute distress and/or prevent harm in emergency situations.
2   Rapid tranquillisation is a five-step process: verbal de-escalation, oral medication, injectable medication, repeat injectable medication, long-acting sedative.
3   Patients who have received rapid tranquillisation medication should receive specialist nursing care following the intervention.
4   Lorazepam is generally considered the safest first-line medication for rapid tranquillisation.
5   Antipsychotic medication should never be used for rapid tranquillisation unless the patient has been previously exposed to antipsychotic treatment and has a normal, current ECG.

ANSWERS TO THE CASE STUDY QUESTIONS

1   Eric is acutely distressed. Additionally, there is a risk both to Eric and to others at the moment. Eric has become threatening towards staff members and his behaviour is unpredictable. He may injure himself if he attacks people or property, and a state of prolonged stress may affect his heart and his blood pressure, making him vulnerable to a further cardiac event. Using rapid tranquillisation would reduce his level of distress and alleviate his prolonged stress levels. It may protect him from becoming involved in an act of violence that may cause harm to himself or to others.

2   Eric has not had any physical health checks or monitoring, meaning that his current physical health state is unknown. He is known to have existing cardiac problems and also has the additional cardiac risk factors of obesity and hypotension.

3   If rapid tranquillisation is given, restraint should be avoided if possible, particularly the prone position, in order to avoid placing pressure on Eric's chest. Eric will need 15-minute physical monitoring for the first hour following rapid tranquillisation, and hourly monitoring following this, until there are no further concerns. If Eric refuses monitoring, you may need to think about whether he needs close observations so that his state of alertness can be continually monitored and any warning signs that he is becoming unwell be identified quickly. Eric's care plan and risk assessment will need to be updated after the intervention, and a consultant review will need to be arranged within 72 hours, together with an immediate medication review. The rapid tranquillisation incident should be documented in his progress notes, alongside completion of an incident form. Both Eric and the team involved in the intervention will require a debrief. Due to the complexities of Eric's physical health and his physical vulnerability, use of non-physical and non-medicinal interventions should also be considered.

4   If a decision was made to give Eric medication for rapid tranquillisation, you would choose to give lorazepam. You would not give aripiprazole. This is because Eric has not had a recent physical health assessment, does not have a recent ECG and has existing cardiac risk factors. Lorazepam would be the safest option.

REFERENCES AND RECOMMENDED READING

Calver, L., Drinkwater, V. and Isbister, G.K. (2013) 'A prospective study of high dose sedation for rapid tranquilisation of acute behavioural disturbance in an acute mental health unit', *BMC Psychiatry*, 13: 225.

Department of Health (2014) 'New drive to end deliberate face-down restraint'. Available online via www.gov.uk/government/publications/positive-and-proactive-care-reducing-restrictive-interventions (accessed 15 October 2021).

Haddad, P. and Anderson, I. (2002) 'Antipsychotic-related QTc prolongation, torsade de pointes and sudden death', *Drugs*, 62 (11): 1649–71.

Loonen, A. and Ivanova, S. (2020) 'Neurobiological mechanisms associated with antipsychotic drug-induced dystonia', *Journal of Psychopharmacology*, 35 (1). https://doi.org/10.1177/0269881120944156.

Mind (2013) Mental Health Crisis Care: Physical Restraint in Crisis. A Report on Physical Restraint in Hospital Settings in England. London: Mind.

Mind (2021) 'Psychiatric medicine'. Available at: www.mind.org.uk/information-support/drugs-and-treatments/medication/drug-names-a-z (accessed 1 October 2021).

Murphy, R. and Wales, P. (2013) *Mental Health Law in Nursing*. London: Learning Matters.

NICE (2015) 'Violence and aggression: Short-term management in mental health, health and community settings', NICE guideline (NG10). Available at: www.nice.org.uk/guidance/ng10 (accessed 26 October 2016).

NICE (2016) 'Psychosis and schizophrenia in children and young people: recognition and management', Clinical guideline (CG155). Available at: www.nice.org.uk/guidance/cg155/chapter/Recommendations#possible-psychosis (accessed 2 July 2021).

NICE: British National Formulary (BNF) (2021) The BNF. Available at: https://bnf.nice.org.uk (accessed 4 November 2021).

Richmond, J.S., Berlin, J.S., Fishkind, A.B., et al. (2012) 'Verbal de-escalation of the agitated patient: Consensus Statement of the American Association for Emergency Psychiatry Project BETA De-escalation Workgroup', *Western Journal of Emergency Medicine*, 13 (1): 17–25.

Rund, D.A., Ewing, J.D., Mitzel, K., et al. (2006) 'The use of intramuscular benzodiazepines and antipsychotic agents in the treatment of acute agitation or violence in the emergency department', *Journal of Emergency Medicine*, 31 (3): 317–24.

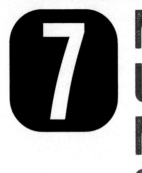

7 MEDICATION USED FOR THE MANAGEMENT OF DEMENTIA

BY SARA SOAMES

AFTER READING THIS CHAPTER, YOU WILL BE ABLE TO:

- Have a basic understanding of dementia
- Be familiar with anti-dementia medications and when they are prescribed
- Be familiar with other psychotropic medications that are used to treat symptoms of dementia
- Have an awareness of the barriers to prescribing medication in dementia

---

WHAT IS DEMENTIA?

'Dementia' can be understood as an umbrella term for a collection of symptoms caused by disease or disorder of the brain. These symptoms are characterised by a decline in a person's **cognitive functioning**, an impairment of the activities of daily living, and/or a change in their behaviour and personality (Waldemar and Burns, 2009).

Dementia is a clinical syndrome and changes to the brain alone are therefore not enough to support a diagnosis; there must be evidence that there has been deterioration in a person's cognitive function and/or ability to engage in activities of daily living. It is not uncommon to find changes to the brain as we age; for instance, those who have vascular or cardiac illnesses are likely to have a degree of small vessel disease that does not impact their cognitive functioning. Sunderland et al. (2007: 11) define clinical syndrome as: 'a constellation of signs and symptoms that, although recognisable in itself, may be attributable to numerous causes of pathological events'.

Most of us will have heard and used the term 'Alzheimer's' but know very little about other types of dementia. The term 'Alzheimer's' dates back to the early 20th century and was named after Dr Alois Alzheimer who, after extensive research, was the first to link symptoms of dementia, such as memory loss, disorientation and visual hallucinations, with damage to the cerebral cortex. Following the death of a patient under his care, he carried out a post-mortem and noted arteriosclerotic changes and senile plaques, in addition to neurofibrillary tangles (Jucker et al., 2006), which are all pathophysiological indicators of Alzheimer's disease. Dementia cannot be properly confirmed until after post-mortem when the brain has been fully examined.

It is estimated that about 800,000 people today have a diagnosis of dementia in the UK, with this figure set to double by 2040. By far the most common form of dementia is Alzheimer's disease (AD), accounting for at least 60 per cent of all dementias; however, this figure is likely to be much greater if we take into account mixed type dementia which is the presence of both AD and vascular dementia (VD) (Julien et al., 2011; Waldemar and Burns, 2009). VD is the second leading cause of dementia and Lewy body dementia (LBD) accounts for around 15–20 per cent of dementia diagnoses (Taylor et al., 2012).

Statistics indicate that the cost of dementia to the UK economy is far higher than that of cancer, heart disease and stroke (Hughes, 2011). As the global population ages, so will the numbers of people diagnosed with dementia increase, with a projection of nearly 75 million cases of dementia estimated to be confirmed worldwide over the next 30 years (World Health Organization, 2017). Dementia is fast becoming the leading cause of mortality worldwide. It is an illness that typically affects the older population; however, it is not a natural part of ageing (Small and Greenfield, 2015). Dementia can also be something that impacts younger people; 'young-onset dementia' is the term we use to refer to those who develop a dementia before the age of 65, and there are currently over 42,000 people in the UK who come into this age bracket (Alzheimer's Society, 2021). These dementias may present differently, with memory-related symptoms appearing later in the presentation, and early symptoms being more around movement and mobility. This form of dementia is more likely to be hereditary (around 10% of cases), a rarer form of dementia and linked to another physical disease.

Adults with a learning disability, in particular those with Down's syndrome, may also be at risk of developing a dementia before the age of 65, in particular Alzheimer's disease. This is because the extra chromosome (chromosome 21) that these individuals are born with carries a gene that produces a protein called APP. This protein then builds up in the brain to develop beta-amyloid plaques, which are known as a hallmark of Alzheimer's dementia. By age 40, more than 50 per cent of people with Down's syndrome will have these plaques and be showing some signs or symptoms, and much more research is needed to understand other risk factors.

We commonly relate dementia with 'forgetfulness', which in the early stages of AD is one the most common symptoms reported (McKeel et al., 2007). However, the symptoms of dementia include language difficulties (both speaking and comprehension), perceptual difficulties, a change to a person's ability to reason, difficulty in processing and retaining information, mood disturbances, decline in the activities of daily living (ADL) function, and visual/auditory hallucinations, to name but a few. Symptoms vary, depending on the type and stage of dementia.

In the UK today, assessment and treatment of the more common forms of dementias – namely AD, VD, mixed type dementia, LBD and frontotemporal dementia (FTD) – tend to fall under secondary mental health services. The purpose of this chapter is to discuss the pharmacological treatments available for the above dementias. However, in order to do this, we must consider and form a good knowledge base of what dementia is, how it affects the brain, how we assess for dementia and, finally, when and what medication would be prescribed. Given the nature of this client group, other factors need to be considered when prescribing medication – for instance, capacity and ability to consent to treatment, family/carer input when prescribing treatment and other medications that can be used to treat symptoms of dementia.

Treatment options are limited for those with a diagnosis of dementia. Anti-dementia medication will not resolve symptoms of cognitive impairment, nor can it stop the progression of dementia. Instead, its main function is to slow down the progression of damage to the brain. Dementia is a progressive illness, meaning that over time damage to the brain will continue to occur and thus symptoms will likely worsen, impacting a person's ability to engage in basic day-to-day tasks such as cooking, cleaning, shopping and taking medication. Dementia may also affect a person's ability to make rational decisions.

Dementia can be a debilitating illness that impacts not only the person themselves, but also their family. In the earlier stages of dementia, families will often report feeling guilty about losing their patience with their loved ones due to symptoms of forgetfulness. They also often find themselves taking on a huge caring role that can impact their own physical and mental health. In some cases where the illness progresses to a stage where the person is not safe to remain at home, relatives may have conflicting views about what is in the best interest of the person:

Dear Dementia,

You've turned my family against one another. I wish they could see it's not WHO'S right it's WHAT'S right that matters.

(From Ian Donaghy, *Dear Dementia*, 2015)

HOW DOES DEMENTIA AFFECT THE BRAIN?

The brain is a hugely complex organ. This chapter will look briefly at how the different parts of the brain regulate certain functions and where in the brain you might find damage. Once again, it is important to stress that computed tomography (CT) or magnetic resonance imaging (MRI) of head scans alone are not to be relied on to form a diagnosis of dementia. The clinical symptoms must fit the diagnostic criteria. The main parts of the brain are (see Figure 7.1):

1   *The brainstem* can be found towards the base of the brain. The brainstem plays an integral part in important functions such as breathing and swallowing, heart rate/blood pressure, and our state of consciousness – i.e. whether we are awake or asleep.

2   *The cerebellum* is formed of two parts, which surround the top of the brainstem. These are key players in receiving messages from our sensory systems and spinal cord. These messages enable the cerebellum to coordinate deliberate movements such as posture, gait, balance and speech.

3   *The cerebrum* is the largest part of the brain and is divided into two hemispheres – the cerebral hemispheres. The right cerebral hemisphere is responsible for functions such as spatial awareness and perception, and the left cerebral hemisphere is responsible for functions that include language and reasoning.

4   *The lobes* are located within the cerebral hemispheres and are known as the occipital lobe, parietal lobe, temporal lobe and frontal lobe. The occipital lobe is responsible for visual information, in other words understanding and processing what our eyes see. The parietal lobe is responsible for the comprehension of language and for perception. The frontal lobes are responsible for judgement, smell, emotions, behaviours and executive function, meaning how we plan, organise and solve problems.

5   *The hippocampus* is a subcortical (below the cortex) structure of the cerebrum. It can be described as the memory centre as it has a key function in shaping new memories of events that we have experienced.

6   *The limbic system* connects the brainstem and cerebral hemispheres together. Its structure includes the hippocampus, which, as mentioned above, is vital in shaping new memories.

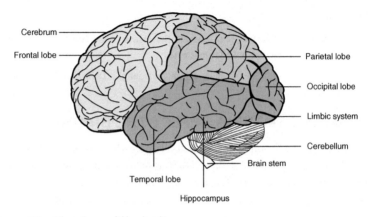

Figure 7.1 Structure of the brain

In the earlier stages of AD, you would typically find **atrophy** (shrinkage) to the hippocampus, and early symptoms include forgetfulness and word-finding difficulties. As the disease progresses, damage to the brain increases and occurs in other parts of the cerebral cortex, affecting a wider range of cognitive functions.

In VD, there would be the presence of small vessel disease across the brain and possibly old infarct; it is not specific to one area. Small vessel disease is the result of narrowing/blocking of small vessels in the brain. It can be caused by a wide range of physical health problems (e.g. hypertension, stroke, heart problems and diabetes). The CT head scan may also show atrophy; however, this can be normal with ageing. Diagnosis of this type of dementia is dependent on the location of atrophy and on the presenting symptoms. People with vascular type dementia often function quite highly in their day-to-day routine, and cognitive testing, presenting symptoms and physical health history are quite important when making this diagnosis.

Mixed type dementias are a combination of different types of dementia, most commonly AD and VD. Due to the combination of changes to the brain, the symptoms and progression can be similar to that of an AD.

In FTD, there tends to be the presence of asymmetrical atrophy to the frontal temporal lobes; however, in many cases CT results do not detect changes. A diagnosis of FTD is largely symptom based. Early symptoms often include changes to the personality, a lack of personal and social awareness, disinhibition, impulsivity and rigid thinking. As this type of dementia typically manifests in people aged 55–65, it can be misdiagnosed as other psychiatric disorders. Memory problems tend to become more apparent in later stages.

LBD may show a degree of atrophy or normal age-related changes; however, as with FTD, more often than not, CT head scanning may not detect changes. Making a diagnosis is dependent on clinical symptoms, for instance visual hallucinations, parkinsonian symptoms, rapid eye movement (REM) sleep disturbance and a decline in cognitive functioning.

Table 7.1 Different types of dementia

Type of dementia	Common changes	Typically affected parts of the brain	Treatment indicated
Alzheimer's in dementia (AD)	Atrophy	Hippocampus, medial temporal area	Yes
Vascular dementia (VD)	Small-vessel disease, atrophy, old infarcts	Non-specific	No
Mixed-type dementia	Small vessel disease, atrophy	Hippocampus, medial temporal area	Yes
Lewy body dementia (LBD)	Normal Age-related changes	Clumps of proteins (Lewy bodies) inside brain cells Can only be detected with position emission tomography (PET scan)	Yes
Frontotemporal dementia (FTD)	Atrophy	Frontal and anterior temporal lobes Widening of the frontal ventricular system	No

Note: The treatment indicated field refers specifically to anti-dementia medication and does not include the use of antipsychotic medication or antidepressants.

For more information on the symptoms of dementia, see the Alzheimer's Society website at: www.alzheimers.org.uk

WHEN DO WE PRESCRIBE ANTI-DEMENTIA MEDICATIONS?

Anti-dementia medication is prescribed following a diagnosis of dementia. Before this diagnosis is given, a full physical health screening, comprehensive cognitive assessment and CT head scan are recommended (NICE, 2006). This is not only to rule out physical or other psychiatric causes that may impact a person's cognitive functioning but also to ascertain whether pharmacological treatments are appropriate.

In certain cases, anti-dementia medication will be prescribed without a CT head scan. This may be because the person is unable to attend a CT scan due to age or mobility and their presenting symptoms are assessed to be directly related to a specific type of dementia, or because the person lacks the capacity to make decisions regarding treatment and the responsible clinician has decided that it is in their best interest to start treatment.

Undiagnosed and poorly managed physical health conditions such as infection, stroke, **atrial fibrillation**, **hypothyroidism**, **hyperthyroidism**, irregular sodium levels (**hyponatraemia/hypernatraemia**) and diabetes can cause cognitive decline and possible misdiagnosis of dementia. It is important to know the patient's physical health history and ensure that symptoms are not being caused or exacerbated by physical health problems. This is a patient group who are generally older and therefore more likely to have pre-existingphysical health issues that may impact their cognitive ability.

Dementia-screening bloods and **urinalysis** are a routine part of assessment and should include: full blood count (FBC), erythrocyte sedimentation rate (ESR), C-reactive protein (CRP), urea and electrolytes (U&Es), liver function test (LFTs), thyroid-stimulating hormone (TSH), serum vitamin B12 and folate, and glucose.

Medication such as analgesia, steroids, psychotropics (antidepressants, antipsychotics and **anxiolytics**) and anticholinergics can also impact a person's cognitive functioning. Another factor to consider is alcohol or substance misuse, both of which can impact cognitive functioning and mimic symptoms of cognitive impairment, such as confusion, disorientation, reduced appetite and forgetfulness. Long-term alcohol abuse in some cases can cause an alcohol-related dementia known as Wernicke–Korsakoff syndrome.

A very important condition to mention when discussing dementia is delirium. Research indicates that the older population (>65) are at the greatest risk of developing a delirium (Cole et al., 2009). Delirium is one of the most common causes for confusion in older adults and can manifest similarly to a dementia; it can be best described as an organic mental confusion which fluctuates in its nature (Schroeder, 2017). Often misdiagnosed as a dementia or other psychiatric disorder due to the similarity in symptoms (Johnson, 2001), people can present as agitated, experience visual hallucinations, express bizarre thoughts and perceptions, and experience a marked decline in cognitive function. The onset is generally rapid, with a change to a person's mental state being seen within hours or days (Bracewell et al., 2005). There are many precipitating factors for delirium: systemic infection, metabolic disturbance, vitamin deficiency, endocrine disease, intracranial difficulties, complication post surgery or dementia (Kumar and Clark, 2002; NHS Evidence, 2012). When left untreated, delirium can develop into a dementia.

Cognitive assessments serve several purposes. First, they give the clinician an idea of the types of symptoms that a person may be experiencing and onset of symptoms. Second, they enable clinicians to carry out cognitive testing that determines whether a person's level of cognition is indicative of a dementia and whether they require further investigations, such as a CT head scan or neuropsychological testing. Third, they help to rule out other psychiatric conditions that can sometimes mimic a dementia – for instance depression and anxiety. People with low mood and anxiety can often present with poor concentration that may result in forgetfulness, apathy, reduced appetite, tiredness or insomnia, all symptoms that, when treated with anti-depressants/anxiolytics, may resolve. And, finally, they help to find out how the person manages in their day-to-day life, for instance physical health issues, activities of daily living and medication management, which are all important factors when prescribing medication and monitoring compliance in the future.

There is a wide range of cognitive tests available for use in dementia assessment. Deciding on which test to use is largely dependent on your clinic setting – for instance, GPs and acute general hospitals may use a shorter cognitive test such as the General Practitioner assessment of Cognition (GPCOG) or the Abbreviated Mental Test (AMT) and refer to more specialist services, such as memory assessment services, if cognitive impairment is indicated.

The three main tests used when assessing dementia are the Standardised Mini-Mental State Examination (SMMSE), the Montreal Cognitive Assessment (MOCA) and the Addenbrooke's Cognitive Examination (ACE III). Both the SMMSE and MOCA are scored out of 30, and generally a score lower than 26 is indicative of cognitive impairment. However, this is where your collateral information comes in handy. For instance, if someone did not obtain a basic education or suffers from dyslexia, you might want to take that into account; conversely where someone is highly educated, they might score higher in these tests. Generally, losing points in recall (recalling the words that you asked them to remember) is an indicator of a dementia. The ACE III is a slightly longer test and scored out of 100. This may be a good test to use if someone is highly educated or their memory-loss symptoms are milder; scores below 90 are generally indicative of a cognitive impairment and may require further investigation.

Following assessment if indicated, the patient will be referred for a CT head/MRI scan. This detects whether there are changes to the brain that are related to a dementia and whether treatment is appropriate.

THE MEDICINES LIST

There are two groups of medications used specifically for the treatment of dementia: acetylcholinesterase inhibitors and N-methyl-D-aspartate (NMDA) receptor antagonists.

Acetylcholinesterase inhibitors

Acetylcholinesterase inhibitors (often shortened to cholinesterase inhibitors) are prescribed for people with AD, mixed type or LBD. In healthy brains, acetylcholine is broken down by an enzyme called acetylcholinesterase (AchE). Acetylcholine is very important as it is a neurotransmitter (neurotransmitters send signals between brain cells). In cases of AD, mixed type or LBD, there is a lack of acetylcholine, which means that signals are not being sent to other cells, resulting in cognitive impairment. Acetylcholinesterase inhibitors prevent the action of acetylcholinesterase, which in turn raises the level of acetylcholine in the brain and therefore slows down the progression of cognitive decline. There is also evidence to suggest that cholinesterase inhibitors can be effective in treating behavioural problems that are related to dementia and that they may have beneficial psychotropic effects in patients with AD – for instance, improve mood and reduce apathy (Cummings, 2000; Hopker, 1999). In addition, certain types of cholinesterase inhibitors have other mechanisms of action that can help with cognitive functioning. Prior to starting this medication, the person's pulse rate and weight should be taken; both should be monitored regularly because this type of medication can cause bradycardia and weight loss.

These types of medications do not cause dependency. Commonly seen side effects include dizziness, nausea, diarrhoea, fatigue, insomnia, agitation and bradycardia. Less common side effects include atrioventricular (AV) block in the heart, seizures, gastric and duodenal ulcers.

Acetylcholinesterase inhibitors interact with the following medicines:

- *Fluvoxamine*: Affects the metabolism of cholinesterase inhibitors which can lead to increased levels of in cholinesterase inhibitors in blood
- *Tricyclic medication (e.g. Amitryptaline)*: Cholinesterase inhibitors increase cholinergic effects, tricylcic medication decreases cholinergic effect
- *Beta blockers, calcium channel blockers, and antiarrhythmic medication*
- *Anticholinergic medication*: Reduces the efficacy of cholinesterase inhibitors; anticholinergic medication should be stopped with caution
- *Theophylline*: Cholinesterase inhibitors increase the level of theophylline in the blood, which can potentially be fatal
- *Smoking (tobacco)*: Reduces the level of cholinesterase inhibitor in the blood

Drug name: **Donepezil** – usually the first-line treatment for mild to moderate AD or mixed type dementia

UK brand names: Aricept, Aricept Evess (orodispersible)

Average doses: The starting dose for donepezil is generally 5mg once daily. If there are no side effects then it can be increased to 10mg after six to eight weeks. For patients who are elderly, underweight, frail or have severe cardiac conditions, 2.5mg once daily or 5mg on alternate days may be more appropriate

What form does it come in? Tablet, orodispersible tablet

Does it interact with any other medicines? Yes, when taken with beta blockers, risk of brachycardia can increase

Drug name: **Rivastigmine** – used for the treatment of mild to moderate AD, mixed type dementia and LBD. Rivastigmine also works on butyrylcholinesterase (BuChE), another cholinesterase enzyme

UK brand names: Exelon

Average doses:

- Starting dose for tablets and liquid solution: 1.5mg twice daily (bd), which can be increased in two-week intervals where there are no side effects
- Maximum daily dose for tablets and liquid: 6mg bd

(Continued)

- Starting dose for transdermal patches: 4.6mg/24-hour patch, once daily for a minimum of four weeks. Where there are no side effects, this can be increased to 9.5mg/24-hour patch

What form does it come in? Tablet, liquid and transdermal patch

Does it interact with any other medicines? Yes, when taken with beta blockers, risk of brachycardia can increase

---

Drug name: **Galantamine**

UK brand names: Reminyl, Reminyl XL, Acumor XL, Galsya XL

Average doses: Galantamine is available in both immediate release and modified release (XL) tablets. The starting dose for immediate release tablets and liquid form is 4mg twice daily (bd) for at least four weeks. If there are no side effects, then this can be increased to 8mg bd for at least a further four weeks. If no side effects are experienced following the increase, the **maintenance dose** is usually 8-12mg bd. For galantamine XL, the starting dose is 8mg once daily (od) for at least four weeks. If there are no side effects, then this can be increased to 16mg od for at least a further four weeks. If no side effects are experienced following the increase, then the maintenance dose is usually 16-24mg od

What form does it come in? Immediate/modified release (XL) tablet/liquid

Does it interact with any other medicines? Yes, when taken with beta blockers, risk of brachycardia can increase

N-methyl-D-aspartate (NMDA) receptor antagonists

NMDA receptor antagonists work by protecting brain cells from excess glutamate by acting as an antagonist at the NMDA receptor. Glutamate is another chemical that helps to send messages between nerve cells. When the brain is damaged by Alzheimer's, glutamate is released at an excessive rate. Until recently, memantine has been used to treat moderate to severe Alzheimer's. However, results from randomised controlled trials have now shown that prescribing memantine with a cholinesterase inhibitor has had good outcomes for improving cognitive functioning (Atri et al., 2013).

This type of medication is not addictive. Side effects commonly seen include constipation, dizziness and drowsiness. Less common side effects include breathing difficulties, headache and hypertension.

Drug name: Memantine – is used for the treatment of moderate to severe AD and mixed type dementia or where cholinesterase inhibitors have not been tolerated

UK brand names: Exiba

Average doses: The starting dose is 5mg once daily (od) for at least six weeks. If there are no side effects, then this can be increased to 20mg od; however, increasing by 5mg intervals is recommended to monitor for side effects. For patients with impaired renal function, who are prescribed other dementia medication or are frail, starting at 5mg may be more appropriate

What form does it come in? Tablet and liquid

Does it interact with any other medicines? Yes. The following interactions are known:

- Trimethoprim: May increase memantine levels in blood
- Trihexyphenidyl: May cause dizziness, dry mouth and urinary retention

Antipsychotic medication used to treat symptoms of dementia

Antipsychotic medication can be used to treat behavioural and psychological symptoms of dementia (BPSD). These symptoms, such as agitation, aggression, restlessness, poor sleep and visual/auditory hallucinations, can occur in the later stages of dementia. They can be extremely frightening and disturbing for both the patient and their family/carers. It is important to ascertain whether the onset of these symptoms is a sign of their dementia or is caused by other factors. Physical health issues such as constipation, pain, infection and dehydration can all cause the symptoms mentioned above. NICE (2015a) recommends that in addition to monitoring physical health, a thorough home environment assessment is carried out in order to identify

(Continued)

any external stimulus or triggers that may have caused or be contributing to the onset of symptoms. When carrying out these assessments, the person's ability to communicate must be taken into account – for instance, they may experience difficulties with language or processing information and as a result may not be able to verbalise what is causing them distress.

Using antipsychotics to treat BPSD must be done with caution and as a last resort; it is advisable to carry out an ECG on the patient or at the earliest possible opportunity prior to starting antipsychotic medication. The two recommended antipsychotics used to treat BPSD are risperidone and quetiapine. Typical (first-generation) antipsychotics are generally not appropriate for use in BPSD as their side effect profile is much larger. Side effects include parkinsonian symptoms such as stooped posture, shuffled gait, stiffness and slowness when moving. Other side effects include constipation, oversedation and higher levels of confusion, which in turn can increase a person's risk of falls and deterioration to mental state. Haloperidol at a low dose (0.5-1.5mg) is sometimes used to treat BPSD; however, it is not recommended due to side effects such as involuntary facial movements around the mouth area (tardive dyskinesia), which is often irreversible. Haloperidol is generally used within an acute medical setting to treat symptoms of delirium.

Drug name: **Haloperidol**

UK brand names: Dozic, Haldol, Serenace

Average doses: 0.5-1.5mg

- IM injection: 2-5mg daily

What form does it come in? Tablet, capsule, liquid, emergency injection, depot injection (depot injection is not appropriate for use in BPSD in dementia)

Does it interact with any other medicines? Yes. Please refer to pp. 130-31

Drug name: **Risperidone**

NICE guidelines and the British National Formulary recommend using risperidone for BPSD in AD; however, it can also be used to treat BPSD in VD and FTD. The starting dose should ideally be as low as possible – i.e.

250mcg once daily (od) and no more than 1mg twice daily (bd). To note, the lowest tablet form is 500mcg: if a patient is prescribed lower than this (i.e. 250mcg) the tablet will need to be cut in half

UK brand names: Risperdal, Risperdal Consta (depot)

Average doses: 250mcg–2mg daily

What form does it come in? Tablet, liquid and depot injection (depot injection is not appropriate for use in BPSD in dementia)

Does it interact with any other medicines? Yes. Please refer to p. 134

For BPDS, or where psychotic symptoms are persistent and distressing in LBD, the recommended treatment is quetiapine as the parkinsonian side effects are lower. Starting dose is recommended at 25mg; however, this will depend on the severity of symptoms, physical health, weight and frailty. Starting at 12.5mg and increasing slowly if no side effects are apparent may be more appropriate. Modified release versions are not appropriate for treating BPSD. To note, the lowest tablet form is 25mg; if a patient is prescribed lower than this (i.e. 12.5mg) the tablet will need to be cut in half

***Drug name*: Quetiapine**

UK brand names: Atrolak, Biquelle, Ebesque, Seroquel, Tenprolide, Zaluron

Average doses: 12.5mg–100mg

What form does it come in? Tablet only

Does it interact with any other medicines? Yes. Please refer to pp. 106–07

Antidepressant medication used to treat symptoms of dementia

Symptoms of depression are often reported or apparent in people who suffer from dementia. Where this is the case, treating these symptoms with antidepressant medication may be indicated; like all medications

(Continued)

prescribed for older adults, this needs to be done with caution and monitored carefully. Medication should be started at the lowest dose and increased slowly to monitor for side effects. Tricyclic and mono-amine oxidase inhibitor (MAOIs) are not recommended for use in symp-toms of depression in dementia due to their high side effect profile. SSRIs (sertraline and citalopram) and SSNIs (mirtazapine) are preferable treatment options. As with all antidepressants, the type of medication prescribed is dependent on symptoms. For instance, if someone is expe-riencing poor sleep and reduced appetite, then mirtazapine may be a good choice at lower doses as it has a sedating effect and increases appetite. Sertraline works well with people who may be presenting with apathy as it has a less sedating effect. Sertraline or citalopram may be a good choice if a person is prescribed an antipsychotic for BPSD because antipsychotic medications are sedating.

Drug name: Citalopram

UK brand names: Cipramil

Average doses: 10–20mg

What form does it come in? Oral drops and tablet

Does it interact with any other medicines? Yes, please refer to pp. 13–14

Note: Calculating a citalopram oral drop dose is slightly different to other liquid preparations: four drops equate to 8mg, which is the therapeutic equivalent of a 10mg tablet.

Drug name: Sertraline

UK brand names: Lustral

Average doses: 25–100mg daily

What form does it come in? Tablet only

Does it interact with any other medicines? Yes. Please refer to pp. 16–17

Note: If a person is prescribed 25mg, then this medication will need to be cut in half.

Drug name: **Mirtazepine**

UK brand names: Zispin

Average doses: 7.5–45mg daily

What form does it come in? Tablet, orodispersible tablet and liquid

Does it interact with any other medicines? Yes. Please refer to pp. 17–18

Note: If a person is prescribed 7.5mg, then this medication will need to be cut in half

Other medication used to treat symptoms of dementia

Drug name: **Promethazine hydrochloride** – an antihistamine often used for rapid tranquillisation due to its sedating effect. Promethazine can be prescribed in dementia to reduce symptoms such as agitation, restlessness and insomnia. Administration via intramuscular injection is only appropriate within a ward environment where oral administration has not been effective

UK brand names: Phenergan

Average doses: 10–50mg daily (do not exceed 100mg in 24 hours)

What form does it come in? Tablet, liquid and intramuscular injection (IM – should be used with caution in BPSD in dementia)

Does it interact with any other medicines? Yes. The following interactions are known:

- *Tricyclics and MAOIs*: Increased antimuscarinic and sedative effect
- Anti-arrhythmic medication and beta blockers: Increased risk of ventricular arrhythmias

Drug name: **Trazodone** – an antidepressant sometimes used with dementia to treat BPSD, anxiety or agitation due to its sedating effect. The starting dose to treat symptoms of BPSD, anxiety or agitation is usually 25mg

(Continued)

once daily (od) and should not exceed 100mg in 24 hours; increasing the dose should be done with caution due to its sedating effect.

UK brand names: Trazodone hydrochloride

Average doses: 25-100mg od

What form does it come in? Tablet, capsule and liquid

Does it interact with any other medicines? Yes. The following interactions are known:

- *Amitriptyline*: Increases the risk of developing serotonin syndrome
- *Tramadol*: Increases the risk of developing serotonin syndrome and may increase the risk of seizures - unrelated to serotonin syndrome

***Drug name:* Lorazepam** - Lorazepam is a benzodiazepine often used for rapid tranquillisation and management of symptoms of anxiety due to its sedating effects. Benzodiazepines are not generally recommended for use in dementia; however, where someone is in an acute phase of their illness, it may be necessary. It is available in tablet, liquid and injection form. Administration via intramuscular injection is only appropriate within a ward environment where oral administration has not been effective

UK brand names: Ativan

Average doses:

- Oral: 0.5-1mg
- IM injection: 0.5-1mg
- Total maximum within 24 hours: 2mg

What form does it come in? Tablet, solution for emergency injection

Does it interact with any other medications: Yes. Please refer to p. 47

Drug name: Melatonin – used to treat sleep disorders. This medication can have good effect in managing insomnia in people with dementia, though at the time of publication draft NICE guidelines do not recommend using melatonin for supporting sleep disturbance in people with dementia. At present, it is only licensed for use at 2mg at night in dementia; however if advised by a sleep specialist then there is the potential to increase to 4mg at night

UK brand names: Circadin

Average doses: 1–2mg

What form does it come in? Tablet only

Does it interact with any other medicines? Yes. The following interactions are known:

- *Fluvoxamine*: Increases the level of melatonin in blood
- *Vemurafenib*: Increases the level of melatonin in blood

Drug name: Pregabalin – generally used to treat peripheral and central neuropathy; however, it has very good outcomes for treating anxiety (doses will be different). The starting dose is usually 25mg once daily (od), it should be increased at 25mg increments and should not exceed 600mg in a 24-hour period

UK brand names: Lyrica

Average doses: 25mg–300mg

What form does it come in? Tablet and liquid

Does it interact with any other medicines? Yes. The following interactions are known:

- *Buprenorphine*: Both drugs act on the central nervous system – used together they may cause respiratory depression and coma fatality

CONSENT TO TREATMENT AND MAKING CAPACITOUS DECISIONS

Most people with a diagnosis of dementia will be able to make informed and capacitous decisions about their care and treatment. However, those who are in an acute or later stage of their illness may lack capacity to make decisions; this may be related to treatment, the type of support they need, or where they live. Family and carer input is very important in these circumstances. Their opinions are invaluable as they will have a greater knowledge about the person's wishes, needs and preferences. Some people may have completed advanced directives or statements that can be used as a guide when making decisions.

Those who require inpatient admission but lack capacity to consent to admission and treatment sometimes require assessment under the Mental Health Act 1983. Patients who are detained in hospital under the Act may need some form of treatment; however, in certain cases, administering medication can prove difficult if the patient refuses it and they lack capacity to understand why treatment may be necessary and are unlikely to regain capacity.

Where this is the case, covert medication can be used. 'Covert medication' refers to medication administered without the patient knowing; this may be in food or drink (NICE, 2015b). In order to use covert medication legally, there must be evidence that covertly administering the said medication is in the patient's best interest and that other routes of medication administration have been trialled. In addition, a capacity test (discussed later) must be completed, and the patient's family or representative must agree and sign the covert medication form, which must also be signed by the responsible clinician, a registered nurse and a pharmacist. All medications that are intended to be covertly administered must be listed on this form; medication that is not listed on the form must not be covertly administered as this would be illegal. Covert medication can be administered both under the MHA 1983 and the Mental Capacity Act (MCA) 2005.

FACT BOX 7.1

Some medications cannot be mixed with certain food/drink products as they change the mechanism of action. Always check with a pharmacist.

Once treatment has been established with good effect, if the person continues to lack capacity, then they may no longer require detention under the MHA 1986. In these circumstances, it may be more appropriate to use the MCA 2005. Deprivation of Liberty Safeguard (DoLS) falls under the MCA 2005. This is a legal framework that safeguards vulnerable people who lack capacity to make decisions in their best interest. It is much less restrictive than the MHA 1986 and can be used within a care home setting.

Capacity as a general rule is specific and related to a particular decision at a particular time (Mental Capacity Act 2005) and it should therefore be assessed regularly. The MCA 2005 assumes that all people have capacity to make decisions until assessed otherwise. In certain situations, a person may be deemed to permanently lack capacity – that is, they have a progressive brain disorder or disability. Where capacity has been identified as a concern, a four-point test is carried out. If one or more of the following conditions from the test is not met, then that person will be deemed to lack capacity:

1   Is the person able to understand the information relevant to the decision?
2   Is the person able to retain that information?
3   Is the person able to weigh up that information as part of the process of making a decision?
4   Is the person able to communicate their decision (whether by talking, using sign language or any other means)?

Note: It is important that this test is strictly related to how the decision is made and not the outcome.

LEARNING FROM A CASE STUDY: TEST YOUR KNOWLEDGE

Case Study 7.1

Mr Herbert is a 79-year-old man who has recently been diagnosed with dementia in Alzheimer's mixed type. He has been prescribed donepezil 5mg. You have been allocated to see Mr Herbert to monitor his response to treatment. You read through his initial assessment prior to meeting him and note that he mentioned that he was forgetting to take his medication:

1   What would you consider during the review?

(Continued)

Mr Herbert reports that since starting donepezil 5mg, he has experienced loose stools, which, in turn, has resulted in a decrease in his appetite. He does not want to eat too much as he is scared that he might soil himself. You take his pulse rate, which reads 52 (a 9-beat decrease from the initial assessment).

2   What advice would you give Mr Herbert?
3   What information would you feed back to the MDT?

Case Study 7.2

Mrs Khan is an 86-year-old woman who lives with her family. She has a diagnosis of Lewy body dementia, for which she is prescribed rivastigmine 9.6mg transdermal patches and quetiapine 12.5mg twice daily (bd). Some of her symptoms include visual hallucinations, agitation and restlessness, which she finds very distressing. Her symptoms are complicated by frailty and poor mobility. Physical causes have been ruled out as the cause of current symptoms. She was detained under section 2 of the Mental Health Act as her family were struggling to manage her symptoms. She has been on the ward for a week, her symptoms have not improved and she continues to experience visual hallucinations and agitation. Her sleep is poor and she is restless, particularly at night. During the weekly MDT, it was decided to increase quetiapine to 25mg at night, whilst the morning dose was to remain at 12.5mg:

4   What would you assess for with this increase to medication?
5   What are the risks associated with this increase to medication?

IF I REMEMBER 5 THINGS FROM THE CHAPTER...

1   Dementia is a clinical syndrome. This means that a diagnosis is based on *symptoms* as well as pathophysiology.
2   There are two types of anti-dementia medications: cholinesterase inhibitors and NMDA receptor antagonists. They work by slowing down the progression of symptoms that occur in dementia.
3   When monitoring the response to cholinesterase inhibitors, weight and pulse must be monitored.
4   Antipsychotic medication used to treat BPSD should always be a last resort and must be reviewed every 12 weeks.
5   Where possible, family and carer input should always be sought when making decisions about treatment.

ANSWERS TO THE CASE STUDY QUESTIONS

Case Study 7.1

1 Consider whether he has been remembering to take his medication (check the number of tablets if you are not sure) and if he has noted any side effects, for instance loose stools/stomach upset, reduced appetite. Checking his weight and pulse is also recommended.

2 Ask Mr Herbert whether the loose stools started around the same time as he started on his medication and whether the decrease to his appetite is physical or psychological. Check whether there has been any significant weight loss. Ensure that he has been taking medication so as to ensure that the symptoms are related to the medication and not physical illness. If so, advise Mr Herbert to stop taking the medication, inform him that donepezil can sometimes cause loose stools. Explain that there are alternative medications to donepezil. Offer to review him the following week in order to assess whether the symptoms have resolved.

3 Feed back to the nurse in charge what Mr Herbert reported and your own concerns regarding the loose stools and lowered pulse. Explain the advice that you gave him and your rationale.

Case Study 7.2

4 You would assess whether there has been a response to treatment. Has there been an improvement to Mrs Khan's symptoms? Is she less agitated? Has her sleep improved? Does she continue to experience visual hallucinations? Have you noticed any side effects: stiffness, hypersalivation, oversedation? Has her mobility worsened? Have there been any falls or near falls since increasing medication?

5 Increased risk of stroke is strongly associated with antipsychotic medication, although less so with quetiapine. There is an increased risk of falls with this type of medication due to its sedating effect. Arrhythmia (problem with the heart rhythm) is associated with quetiapine. Taking or repeating an ECG as early as possible is recommended.

REFERENCES AND RECOMMENDED READING

Alzheimer's Society (2021) 'Young-onset dementia'. Available at www.alzheimers.org.uk/about-dementia/types-dementia/younger-people-with-dementia#content-start (accessed 5 July 2021).

Atri, A., Molinuevo, L.J., Lemming, O., et al. (2013) 'Memantine in patients with Alzheimer's disease and receiving donepezil: New analyses of efficacy and safety for combination therapy', *Alzheimer's Research & Therapy*, 5 (1):6.

Bracewell, C., Gray, R. and Gurcharan, R. (2005) *Essential Facts in Geriatric Medicine*. Oxford: Radcliffe Publishing.

Cole, M., Ciampi, A., Beilzile, E. and Zhong, L. (2009) 'Persistent delirium in older hospital patients: A systematic review of frequency and prognosis', *Age and Ageing*, 38 (1): 19–26.

Cummings, J.L. (2000) 'Cholinesterase inhibitors: A new class of psychotropic compounds', *American Journal of Psychiatry*, 157 (1):4–15.

Dickerson, B. and Atri, A. (2014) *Dementia: Comprehensive Principles and Practice*. New York: Oxford University Press.

Donaghy, I. (2015) *Dear Dementia: The Laughter and the Tears*. London: Hawker Publications.

Hopker, S. (1999) *Drug Treatments and Dementia*. London: Jessica Kingsley Publishers.

Hughes, J. (2011) *Alzheimer's and Other Dementias*. Oxford: Oxford University Press.

Johnson, M. (2001) 'Assessing confused patients', *Journal of Neurology, Neurosurgery and Psychiatry*, 71 (Suppl. 1):i7–i12.

Jucker, M., Beyreuther, K., Hass, C., et al. (2006) *Alzheimer: 100 Years and Beyond*. Berlin and Heidelberg: Springer-Verlag.

Julien, M.R., Advokat, D.C. and Comaty, E.J. (2011) *A Primer of Drug Action: A Comprehensive Guide to the Actions, Uses, and Side Effects of Psychoactive Drugs*, 12th edn. New York: Worth Publishers.

Kumar, P. and Clark, M. (2002) *Clinical Medicine*, 5th edn. London: Elsevier Science.

McKeel, D. Burns, J., Meuser, T., et al. (2007) *Alzheimer's Disease*. Oxford: Atlas Medical Publishing.

NHS Evidence (2012) *Delirium: Evidence Update April 2012. A Summary of Selected New Evidence Relevant to NICE Clinical Guideline 103 'Delerium: Diagnosis, Prevention and Management' (2010)*. Manchester: NICE. Available at: www.nice.org.uk/guidance/cg103/evidence/evidence-update-pdf-134649181 (accessed 1 October 2021).

NICE (2006) 'Dementia: Supporting people with dementia and their carers in health and social care', *NICE Clinical Guideline CG42*. London: NICE.

NICE (2015a) 'Low-dose antipsychotics in people with dementia', NICE Key Therapeutic Topic (KTT7). London: NICE.

NICE (2015b) 'Medicines management in care homes', NICE Quality Standard QS85. London: NICE.

NICE: British National Formulary (BNF) (2021) The BNF. Available at: https://bnf.nice.org.uk (accessed 4th November 2021).

NIH: National Institute for Ageing (2020) 'Alzheimer's disease in people with Down syndrome'. Available at: www.nia.nih.gov/health/alzheimers-disease-people-down-syndrome (accessed 5 July 2021).

Schroeder, K. (2017) *The 10-Minute Clinical Assessment*, 2nd edn. Chichester: John Wiley.

Small, G.W. and Greenfield, S. (2015) 'Current and future treatments for Alzheimer's disease', *American Journal of Geriatric Psychiatry*, 23 (11):1101–5.

Sunderland, T., Jeste, D.V., Baiweyu, O., et al. (eds) (2007) *Diagnostic Issues in Dementia: Advancing the Research Agenda for DSM-V*. Arlington, VA: American Psychiatric Association.

Taylor, D., Paton, C. and Kumar, S. (2012) *The South London and Maudsley NHS Foundation Trust Oxleas NHS Foundation Trust: Prescribing Guidelines in Psychiatry*, 11th edn. Chichester: Wiley-Blackwell.

Waldemar, G. and Burns, A. (2009) *Alzheimer's Disease*. Oxford: Oxford University Press.

World Health Organization (WHO) (2016) *International Classification of Diseases and Related Health Problems, Tenth Edition (ICD-10)*. Geneva: WHO.

World Health Organization (WHO) (2017) *Global Action Plan on the Public Health Response to Dementia 2017–2025*. Geneva: WHO.

APPENDIX

DRUG CALCULATIONS

So, now you have read through all of the chapters, you should have a pretty good idea of the medicines that we use in mental health settings.

Whilst it is essential to understand the different types of medicines and their uses, this knowledge needs to be translated into the care and treatment that we provide as nurses. When we give medication, it is important for us to be able both to understand and to explain what the medicine is for, and that we can safely calculate the correct dose of medication.

The key formula that you need to remember when completing drug calculations is:

Tablets:

$$\frac{\text{Amount prescribed}}{\text{Amount in a tablet}} = \text{Number required}$$

For example, Jayne is prescribed citalopram 20mg. The tablets are available in 10mg tablets:

Therefore:

$$\frac{\text{20mg (amount prescribed)}}{\text{10mg (amount in a tablet)}} = 2 \text{ tablets}$$

The nurse needs to give 2 × 10mg tablets to Jayne in order for her to receive the correct dose of 20mg.

If you are working with liquid medications, you should also be aware of the following formula:

Dosage calculations:

$$\frac{\text{Amount you want}}{\text{Amount you have}} \times \text{Volume it's in} = \text{Required drug dose}$$

Therefore:

$$\frac{500mg}{200mg} \times 1ml = 2.5ml$$

Example drug calculation scenarios for each chapter discussed in this book will now be provided for you to apply your calculation abilities to your new-found medicines knowledge. The answers can be found at the end of the Appendix (pp. 168–70).

DRUG CALCULATION QUESTIONS

Antidepressants

1 Amy is prescribed 50mg amitriptyline in the morning and a further 75mg amitriptyline at night. She has a supply of 25mg tablets available.

   a How much amitriptyline does Amy take within a 24-hour period if she takes both doses?

   b How many 25mg tablets does Amy need to take for each of her two doses?

2 Walter is currently taking fluoxetine 20mg once daily. The medicine is available in 20mg capsules only.

   a How many capsules should Walter take per day?

3 Patience is prescribed sertraline 50mg, which she takes once a day. Due to a mild swallowing issue, Patience has been prescribed sertraline liquid concentrate instead of tablets. The bottle reads that there is '20mg/1ml'.

   a How many ml should Patience have in her syringe to ensure she has her full dose of 50mg?

   b Sertraline concentrate must always be mixed with another liquid before being taken. The instructions on the bottle read 'Mix the dose with a half cup (4 ounces/120 milliliters) of water, ginger ale, lemon-lime soda, lemonade, or orange juice. Drink all of the mixture immediately.' If Patience takes one dose a day, always with ginger ale, how much ginger ale will she have with her medication in a seven-day week?

Antipsychotics

1 Earl is taking clozapine 350mg daily. This is divided into a dose of 150mg in the morning and 200mg at night. There are 50mg and 100mg tablets available.

a   What is the best (fewest) combination of tablets for Earl to take in the morning?

b   What is the best (fewest) combination of tablets for Earl to take in the evening?

2   Tasha is prescribed a depot of Clopixol (zuclopenthixol decanoate) 500mg, which is due today. The solution available is 200mg/1ml.

a   What is the total volume of solution for injection that should be prepared for Tasha?

3   Bertha is currently starting a new depot injection and is being titrated. Her dosing regime is as follows:

Dose 1 (day 1) 150mg

Dose 2 (day 8) 100mg

a   What is the difference in dose between her first dose and her second dose?

Medicines for managing anxiety

1   Ollie is suffering from acute anxiety. He has been prescribed 10mg diazepam, which he can take when he is feeling very anxious and distressed. Ollie only has 2mg tablets available.

a   How many 2mg tablets should Ollie take to make up his dose of 10mg?

2   Mathilda is currently taking zopiclone to help her sleep at night. Following a recent dose increase, she is prescribed 7.5mg a night. Mathilda only has 3.75mg tablets available.

a   How many 3.75mg tablets should Mathilda take to make up her dose of 7.5mg?

3   Bob uses occasional promethazine when he is feeling very distressed and anxious. He is currently an inpatient and is prescribed 25mg PRN. He is specifically prescribed promethazine syrup rather than tablets, as he has a fear of choking due to his current anxiety. When Bob comes to ask for his PRN you notice the syrup states '6.25mg/5ml'.

a   How many mls do you measure to give Bob his 25mg dose?

Rapid tranquillisation

1   Billy has bipolar disorder and is currently experiencing a manic episode. He is prescribed clonazepam 2mg as a regular medication, four times a day.

a   How much clonazepam does Billy receive in a 24-hour period if he takes each of the four doses?

b   Clonazepam is only available in 0.5mg tablets. How many tablets does he need in order to receive his dose of 2mg?

2   Brenda has schizoaffective disorder and is currently very distressed as she believes that all the food and drink on the ward is poisoned, and that an assassin is trying to kill her. She believes that another person on the ward is the assassin and so she decides to try to fight them for her own protection. In order for you to manage this situation safely, Brenda needs rapid tranquillisation. You are asked to prepare an IM injection of lorazepam 2mg. The lorazepam solution is available in 4mg/1ml and needs to be mixed with distilled water in the ratio 1:1.

a   How much lorazepam do you need to draw up?

b   How much distilled water do you need to draw up?

c   What is the total volume of injection in your syringe?

3   Holly is on a PICU and well known to the ward staff. Holly has schizoaffective disorder. She is 32 years old, has a healthy weight and no other known health conditions. It is therefore decided that when she is highly distressed she is able to have IM haloperidol 2.5mg alongside 25mg promethazine.

a   You are asked to prepare the haloperidol injection, which comes in 5mg/ml. How much do you draw up?

Mood-stabilising medications

1   Florence has bipolar disorder and is currently taking lithium carbonate. Florence currently believes that she cannot swallow properly and has asked for all of her medication to be given to her as liquids. The bottle of lithium liquid available states that the solution is 520mg/5ml. It also states that 'each 5ml contains 520mg of the active substance lithium citrate equivalent to 204mg lithium carbonate'. Florence is prescribed 30ml of lithium liquid per day.

a   How much lithium carbonate is in 5ml of the lithium liquid?

b   How much lithium carbonate is in Florence's 30ml dose?

2   Angelo is currently prescribed 2g of sodium valproate per day. The medicine is available in 500mg tablets.

a   What is 2g in mg?

b   How many 500mg tablets does Angelo need to make up his dose of 2g of sodium valproate?

3   Sam is taking carbamazepine for his bipolar disorder, as he has previously tried lithium and had no response. His current dose is 600mg in the

morning and 600mg in the evening. He asks to see the medication leaflet and notes that this says that 'there is a maximum total dose of 1.6g per day'. He asks you to give him assurance he is receiving less than the total maximum dose per day.

a   Can you give him this assurance?

Medicines for drug and alcohol dependence

1   Tommy is currently prescribed a three-day course of Pabrinex IM (a high-potency vitamin injection) alongside his inpatient detox from alcohol. The IM injection needs to be prepared by mixing two ampoules. One ampoule contains 5ml of solution and the other ampoule contains 2ml of solution.

a   What is the total volume of solution prepared?

2   Mel is currently undergoing a course of opiate substitution therapy. Her next dose of Subutex is prescribed as 16mg. You only have 8mg tablets available.

a   How many Subutex 8mg tablets should you dispense and give to Mel?

Medicines for older people

1   Edna has a diagnosis of vascular dementia. She is currently presenting with some highly distressed behaviours, and so it is decided to give Edna a low dose of 250mcg risperidone. Risperidone tablets are only available in 500mcg tablets.

a   How many 500mcg tablets should you give Edna?

2   Rodney has a moderate stage dementia, and is currently taking memantine 20mg, once per day. Rodney has difficulties swallowing, and so uses memantine liquid. The liquid is available as a 10mg/1ml solution.

a   How much of the oral liquid solution should be given to Rodney to make up his dose of memantine 20mg?

ANSWERS TO DRUG CALCULATION QUESTIONS

Antidepressants

1 a   Amy takes 50mg + 75mg = 125mg amitriptyline per day.

1 b   In the morning, Amy needs to take 25mg × 2 tablets to make up her dose of 50mg. In the evening, she needs to take 25mg × 3 tablets in order to make up her dose of 75mg.

2 a   Walter should take 20mg × 1 fluoxetine capsule daily.

3 a   Patience should have 2.5ml in her syringe.

3 b   Patience will drink 840mls of ginger ale with her medication in a seven-day week.

Antipsychotics

1 a   Earl should take 100mg × 1 tablet and 50mg × 1 tablet to make up his morning dose of 150mg clozapine.

1 b   Earl should take 100mg × 2 tablets to make up his evening dose of 200mg clozapine.

2 a   2.5ml of the 200mg/1ml solution should be drawn up to make Tasha's depot of 500mg Clopixol.

3 a   The difference between dose 1 and dose 2 is 50mg. Dose 2 is 50mg less than dose 1.

Medicines for managing anxiety

1 a   2mg × 5 = 10mg. Ollie should take 2mg × 5 tablets.

2 a   3.75mg × 2 = 7.5mg. Mathilda should take 3.75mg × 2 tablets.

3 a   Bob will need 20ml of promethazine syrup.

Rapid tranquillisation

1 a   8mg in 24 hours.

1 b   4 tablets of 0.5mg = 2mg.

2 a   0.5ml for a 2mg injection.

2 b   0.5ml for a 2mg injection.

2 c   0.5ml + 0.5ml = 1ml injection.

3 a   0.5ml of haloperidol is needed.

Mood-stabilising medications

1 a   204mg.

1 b   1224mg.

2 a   2g = 2000mg.

2 b Angelo needs to take 500mg × 4 tablets to make up his dose of 2g of sodium valproate.

3 a Yes, you can give the assurance. Sam is taking a total of 1200mg per day, which equates to 1.2g and so is under the overall maximum dose.

Medicines for drug and alcohol dependence

1 a 5ml + 2ml = 7ml.

2 a You should give Mel 8mg × 2 tablets to make up her dose of 16mg.

Medicines for older people

1 a 500mcg × 0.5 = 250mcg. This means that you should give Edna half a 500mcg tablet to make up her dose of 250mcg.

2 a Rodney needs 2ml of the oral liquid solution to make up his dose of 20mg.

GLOSSARY

In writing this book, we have tried as much as possible to stay jargon free. However, there may be some terms that you are unfamiliar with. A glossary of useful words (not defined in this book) is provided below.

Remember, when you are working with people in your clinical roles, use whatever words and language that they use. Using people's own words makes things so much more accessible and easier to understand!

Abstinence   To refrain from doing something.

Addiction   A compulsive need for a particular substance or thing, which can be both psychological and physical.

Analgesia   Pain-relieving medication.

Anticholinergic   A medication that inhibits the action of the neurotransmitter acetylcholine.

Anxiolytic   A medication used to reduce anxiety.

Atrial fibrillation   A heart condition that leads to an irregular heartbeat.

Atrophy   The wasting away of a body tissue or organ.

Bradycardia   A slow heartbeat.

Cognitive function   Our abilities in relation to memory, reasoning, attention and language.

Constipation   Finding it hard to empty the bowels.

Delirium   A disturbance of mental functioning that leads to confusion and disorientation.

Dependence   Being reliant on something.

Depot medication   A long-acting medicine that is given through intramuscular injection.

Dorsogluteal site   An intramuscular injection site found in the upper outer quadrant of the buttock.

Dysphoria   Feeling dissatisfied with life.

Euphoria   A feeling of intense happiness and feeling very excited.

Hallucination   An experience in which a person sees something that is not actually present.

Heart palpitation   Feeling like your heart is beating too hard, too fast, missing a beat or fluttering.

Hepatic impairment   A problem with the liver.

Hypernatraemia   High sodium levels.

Hypertension   High blood pressure.

Hyperthyroidism   Overactivity of the thyroid gland.

Hyponatraemia   Low sodium levels.

Hypotension   Low blood pressure.

Hypothyroidism   Underactivity of the thyroid gland.

IM injection   An injection given directly into a muscle (intramuscular).

Impotence   When a man is unable to get an erection and/or unable to orgasm.

Informal patient   A person who is in hospital voluntarily. They are not detained under the Mental Health Act and have the right to refuse treatment and to leave hospital.

Insomnia   Not being able to sleep.

Lethargy   Not having any enthusiasm and feeling like you have no energy.

Maintenance dose   The dose of medicine required to keep a person stable.

Mortality   Death.

Neurotransmitter   A chemical substance that enables communication between brain cells.

Oedema   Swelling.

Polypharmacy   Being prescribed multiple medications.

Postural hypotension   When a person's blood pressure suddenly drops when they move from a lying or sitting position to a standing position.

Psychotropic   A medicine that affects a person's mental state.

Renal impairment   A problem with the kidney.

Respiratory depression   When a person develops very slow breathing, which is inadequate to perform adequate gas exchange.

Sedation   A medicine that calms a person down or helps a person to go to sleep.

Sexual dysfunction   Any difficulties encountered during normal sexual activity.

Tachycardia   Fast heart rate.

Therapeutic dose   The dose of medicine required to produce the required effect for the person.

Urinalysis   A urine test.

Urinary retention   Inability to empty the bladder.

Ventricular fibrillation   A problem with the heart rhythm. The heart beats with rapid, erratic electrical impulses. The ventricles of the heart will not be pumping blood and will quiver uselessly.

Ventrogluteal   A site for IM injections found on the side of your hip.

Vertigo   The sensation that the environment around is moving or spinning.

INDEX